Medical Mythology

Rixta Francis

Published November 2017

Table of contents

Acknowledgements

It's highly risky to mention a lot of names in this section, as you easily hurt someone by forgetting their name. So I stay on the safe side and don't mention anyone.

An exception for my husband Grant, who has always supported me through the process of writing this book and who did the proofreading. And for our dog Merry, who doesn't read books but loves me no matter what I do.

Introduction

Every year trillions[1] of dollars are spent on medical research worldwide. Labs everywhere are filled with people in white coats who work with microscopes and complicated machines. It all looks really impressive and the way these people talk can also give the impression that they are doing really important work. The profession of medical scientist also has high standing in society. But what is really happening? Those trillions of dollars are meant to produce good medical treatments and cures for all kinds of diseases. But these just don't happen. Occasionally something is invented that is really helpful for small groups of people who have congenital disorders or who have been in accidents. But that's it. So what's going on?

Most doctors think that they practise "evidence based medicine", but that's not remotely true. In 2007 the British Medical Journal asked its advisers to answer the question how many generally used medical treatments are supported by good evidence. The results were shocking.
13% is considered beneficial (I'm not sure what is meant with "beneficial")
23% is likely to be beneficial (so not quite proven)
8% is a choice between benefits and harms
6% is unlikely to be beneficial
4% is likely to be ineffective or harmful
46%: effectiveness unknown
Especially the last one should be an eye opener to doctors. And you would assume that these results mean that all of those unproven, or proven to be ineffective, treatments would be abandoned. Or that at least insurance companies would stop covering them. But this investigation was ten years ago and nothing has changed. The same unproven, ineffective and often quite dangerous treatments are still offered to patients on a daily basis all over the world.

But many people still believe that the medical system is great and that cures are just around the corner. They are not. The medical

---

[1] 1 trillion is 1 million x 1 million. Or 1,000,000,000,000. Way more than ordinary people can even imagine.

system is chockfull of flaws and myths and assumptions are everywhere. It's not strange that treatments are so rarely useful.

In my book "The Fiction Of Science" I didn't use any references. Also in this book you won't find a lot of them. A few times I recommend books or websites. But this book is meant to make you think for yourself and do your own research. That is much more useful than me giving you all the information on a silver platter. If you want more information there are hundreds of highly useful books and even more good websites.

A lot of the information in this book is not nice. We have been fooled for a long time and it requires courage to admit that and to change your ideas. I hope this book will help you to separate truth from fiction.

1. A bit of history

Most of us have grown up with the idea that doctors know everything and that you should trust the doctor to know what's best. This idea goes back a long time, but it's a mystery to me how this idea survived all the disasters from the last 200 years. Doctors have convinced themselves and the patients that a medical treatment is good as long as it's "generally accepted practice". But history tells a different story.

Babies were always born at home and though some women died in childbirth most of them survived just fine and infections were rare. But then doctors somehow convinced women in the cities that they should give birth in hospitals, where they would be under the care of qualified doctors instead of midwives. The result was the childbed fever that killed many thousands of women. Dr. Semmelweiss proved that if the doctors washed their hands before delivering the babies the childbed fever disappeared. You would think that all doctors would have welcomed this, but no such thing happened. Also then doctors already had serious trouble admitting that they killed patients and so they went on with their practice for another 20 years, killing many more women.

Bloodletting was a standard practice for some 2000 years. Most doctors did it and were convinced it was beneficial. If they had paid more attention they would have seen that it didn't cure anyone and that many patients died from the treatment. But they kept going on and first in the early 1900's the practice started to disappear.

The smallpox vaccine was dangerous enough in itself, but the damage remained limited when the midwives administered it. But doctors didn't like the competition and demanded that they should only do the vaccinating. From that moment the number of deaths increased rapidly and infections and bad scars became very common.

A common treatment for asthma was arsenic and syphilis was generally treated with mercury. That might be hard to imagine now, but they used to be the standard treatments. Of course many patients died, but that didn't stop doctors from continuing with it. It's only 100 years ago that doctors stopped to prescribe these extremely toxic materials.

Penicillin was discovered in 1928 and very soon it showed that bacteria would get resistant to this drug. But when after the war the drug became pretty easily available doctors started to hand out the injections and pills like they were lollies, even when they knew very well it was useless. For many doctors it became a standard treatment for anything and everything and patients started to expect it. Other antibiotics were developed and they soon became the most prescribed drug category. The problems started to show everywhere. Not only did the bacteria become resistant to the drugs, but they also killed the gut bacteria, which leads to all kinds of health problems. And most antibiotics are quite toxic and side effects can be very serious. You would think that so many years later doctors know this and are very careful with prescribing this stuff. Some are, but many still refuse to see the harm these drugs do. Australian doctors are known to prescribe antibiotics on demand, for anything from a cold to a bronchitis and from a sore finger to a stomachache.

It was common practice to x-ray pregnant women to see if their pelvis was wide enough to give birth naturally. In the 1950's it was proven that this caused leukaemia in the children. But doctors couldn't believe that they caused childhood cancer and so they kept x-raying pregnant women for another 20 years. Nowadays there are warning signs to "notify the staff if you are pregnant before getting the x-ray". The radiation is that dangerous.

During the same period doctors started to prescribe thalidomide to pregnant women for morning sickness. And soon babies were born with deformed arms and legs. It was easy to see the connection, but doctors ignored it and kept prescribing the drug.

In the 1960's it was still common practice that doctors advised their patients to take up smoking, as it was so relaxing. By then research had already indicated that smoking was very unhealthy, but doctors ignored it. And they kept ignoring the connection for a long time. Many of them smoked themselves and nobody objected to doctors being used to advertise cigarettes.
In 1963 Valium came on the market and doctors started prescribing the pills like a miracle treatment for an unhappy life. This way they

created a whole generation of addicted housewives. It didn't take too long before the problems started to show up, but this never stopped doctors from prescribing more and more pills. And I would like to add a line here to state when this practice faded out, but the truth is that it never did. Many doctors still prescribe these kind of pills like they are lollies and still many people get addicted to them.

But let's be honest, there are also doctors who see the dangers of benzodiazepines and they don't prescribe them much anymore. They have simply moved on to the next disaster and prescribe antidepressants to everyone who has troubles in life. Doctors can see that they usually don't work and if they would look at the inserts they would know that these drugs have very dangerous side effects. But that doesn't bother them and they keep prescribing these new miracle pills.

Since the pharmaceutical market exploded doctors are happy to prescribe whatever is available. Many drugs made it on the market, only to be taken off again some years later, because too many patients died. We rarely read about those, but the names are many. Vioxx and Avandia were just two that somehow got media attention. But doctors know about all the drugs that disappeared, because they had to tell their patients that they couldn't prescribe the drugs anymore. But this doesn't stop them from eagerly prescribing new drugs as soon as they come on the market. They even come up with their own ideas to prescribe off label. And they prescribe them to children, even when the drug hasn't been approved for that age group. And they insist that these drugs are safe, for "else they wouldn't be on the market".

It's obvious that doctors are not in the habit of learning from their mistakes or the mistakes from the past. They can see themselves that they help few patients and harm many. They can see that their treatments don't work, but they keep prescribing the same drugs and keep performing the same surgeries that failed them already hundreds of times. So how is it possible that doctors got this reputation that they know everything and help sick people? If anyone knows the answer to this question, please let me know. But whenever you meet a doctor, keep this in mind: "Don't trust me, I'm a doctor". It could save your life.

2. Genes

In the 1850's Gregor Mendel did his famous experiments with plants and noticed that certain characteristics go from one generation to another in a certain pattern. This was the start of genetics and the start of a large number of myths.

Genetic information is stored in genes, but what this means is a mystery. When you look up what genes are chemically you get a long explanation that many people won't quite understand. And though it's interesting, it's not particularly relevant from a medical point of view. A variety of things are attributed to our genes, but in the end these tiny thingies are nothing but a bunch of atoms, just like everything in our body. So how do genes determine what we look like or what are personalities are? That's a guess. Nobody knows and nobody ever will know. Assuming that genes are indeed somehow carriers of genetic information (I assume for now that this is correct) we can only come to the conclusion that genes are the key to life. And nobody has ever been able to describe what exactly life is. And nobody will ever be able to understand that, for it's way beyond the capacity of our human brains. That's also the main problem with the evolution theory: life must have started somewhere, but nobody knows what life is.[2] It just is. And that's also the problem with genes: they just are and nobody can know what they do exactly. But this simple fact has never stopped any researcher to come to wild conclusions about genes and it doesn't stop doctors to blame genes for everything they cannot explain.

In the first part of the 20th century genetic research quickly grew and soon it became the holy grail of medicine. As this kind of research digs into the unknown it sounds so scientific and it so easily impresses people, that the lack of proof is easily overlooked. But once you start looking behind the scientific façade and forget about all the assumptions you see all the things that don't add up.

Mutations
Whether you believe in creation or evolution, it's obvious that the

---

[2] An explanation of the problems with the evolution theory is in chapter 2 of my book The Fiction Of Science.

human race started out with a perfect genome and later we got all the "mutations". Have you ever wondered what a genetic mutation is exactly? What is normal and what is the mutation? It can just as well be that we all have different genes. After all we are all unique. So why the assumption that we should all have the same genes in a different combination? There's no reason for that. There are all kinds of things that cause "mutations" and disease causing genes are usually considered bad mutations. But such bad mutations are very common and considering that the human race has been around for many thousands of years you would assume that there are a lot more and a lot worse. There should be so many bad genes around that after all these thousands of years infertility, miscarriages and stillbirths should have increased enormously, because those bad genes block life. But this hasn't happened and the human race is still going strong.

After nuclear disasters or bombs a lot of disabled children are born and it's always said that the radiation causes damage to the genes. But where is the proof for that? How does the damage occur? What is damage in the genes? How does the damage cause the disabilities? If the radiation causes such a bad damage you would assume that no babies get born at all. But the fertility rates in such areas don't seem to decrease dramatically. There is something wrong in the theory. The radiation is obviously causing damage, but is it in the genes? That's a big question. It could just as well be something at cellular level, with the parents or the baby at conception. Maybe the extreme emotional distress that comes with such disasters has something to do with it? All other options are ignored and all scientists go straight to the genes to look for an explanation.

Genetic diseases

But there are genetic diseases, aren't there? Well, I tend to disagree. At least there is very little evidence to support this theory. If you believe that one faulty gene can cause a certain disease in a person, then this would mean that just one gene is responsible for a huge number of processes in the body. How can that possibly be true? It makes more sense that thousands of genes are equally involved and that something else than a single gene mutation causes the disease. How do genes mutate anyway? They aren't alive in themselves. They are just a bunch of chemicals. So how can something that is not alive mutate? That's an interesting question in itself. Obviously some chemicals in a gene can change, but is that a mutation or just something that happens? And maybe it will also change back again at some point? Nobody does the same genetic test every few years to see if the mutation is still there. So who knows what happens. Maybe the mutation that you have as a child has disappeared when you are an adult. Or it has changed into another mutation. But you might still have the same disease.

Studies have shown that if you take a bunch of cells and you take the nucleus (with all the genes) out the cell won't die, but it will keep functioning perfectly normal. So obviously the genes are not necessary for the normal functioning of the body. If you have a certain disease and all the genetic materials would be removed from all your cells, then you probably would still be sick. How is that possible if the disease is exclusively caused by a gene mutation?

Epigenetics
Epigenetics is the science that looks into the functioning of genes and how we can influence that. The standard theory is that we are the helpless victims of our genes and if we have bad genes that's it. Epigenetics has shown that this is not true. And also a look into history shows that this is not true. A good example is cystic fibrosis, a disease that is solely attributed to one gene mutation. About 1:32 white people have this gene mutation, but 100 years ago this disease was extremely rare and now it's so common that most people have heard about it. Genes don't spread that quickly, so the theory that a gene mutation causes a disease is clearly wrong. Epigenetics has developed the theory that environmental factors are capable of turning genes on and off, which would mean that 100 years ago the CF gene was simply turned off in most people and now it's turned on. If you can find how to turn off these genes you can prevent or cure the disease. It has shown to be true that diseases that are considered to be entirely genetic can be prevented and even cured, though for some reason this research has not made it to the mainstream media.
It all sounds very plausible, but there is a big problem: how do the researchers know that what they do to prevent or cure a disease has something to do with the genes? How do they know that a gene is turned off? Maybe they can see a change in chemicals, but how can

they know what that means? It's all a matter of guesses and assumptions, but facts are missing.

People with Down syndrome have one chromosome triple instead of double and this causes a variety of disabilities. But why does that happen? If genes are so important, then shouldn't an extra chromosome mean that you are a genius, or extremely healthy, or very talented? And why exactly does this triple chromosome cause this specific disability? If you would have just one extra gene from that whole chromosome, would that also cause a disability? Maybe it would cause just one symptom of Down's syndrome? Nobody knows.

Diagnostic problems
I have already explained that having mutated genes doesn't mean you will get a disease. That's also known, for in many cases it's said that a certain gene will only increase your chances to get the disease. If not everyone gets the disease, then obviously the genes can be on or off. But does everyone with a certain disease have the genetic mutation? That is where it gets interesting. If someone would have cystic fibrosis[3] without having the gene, then the whole theory about genetic diseases can go straight into the rubbish bin. So are there people with CF who have a negative genetic test? I tried to find an answer to that question, but quickly bumped into the unshakeable medical paradigm that you cannot have CF if you don't have two of the genes. This simply means that if there would be a patient with all the symptoms of CF, but without the positive genetic test, then the doctor would simply rule out CF and diagnose something else. This way the theory will always be correct, no matter how incorrect it might be. And this will go for all diseases that are said to be solely caused by a genetic mutation. So I don't think we can ever know for sure if this theory is correct or not.

When it's already impossible to say with certainty that a genetic disease exists, then what do we do with a genetic predisposition to a disease? I have no idea how researchers determine what gene is responsible for this predisposition, but it must be a wild guess. Many

---
[3] I keep using cystic fibrosis as an example because it's a common disease that is said to be 100% caused by genes: if you don't have the genes you won't get the disease.

people with the gene won't get the disease and many others with the disease don't have the gene. Quite often the numbers are all over the place and nevertheless the researchers stick with their theory that certain genes increase the chance for a certain disease. A whole industry of genetic testing is based on this. People are scared into getting surgery or other dangerous treatments based on a certain test, which doesn't mean anything.

I know about people who think they are predisposed to something because they have a gene mutation that some 40% of the humans have. How can something ever be a mutation when so many people have it? It's much more likely that this is simply a part of the human genome. Some people have it and some don't. We are all different, so that makes perfect sense. If you start testing people with a certain disease to see if they have this gene mutation, then about 40% of them will have it. This doesn't mean anything whatsoever. Many others with the same disease will test negative. But this kind of mythology is presented to the public as scientific facts. And because people so much like to know why they have got sick these kinds of fantasies get widely accepted.

Genetic research
But genetic research has some results, doesn't it? GMO crops have some resistance against insects and diseases. So the researchers must at least know a bit what they are doing. Wrong. All they do is experimenting and if you do enough experiments you likely will at some point find something that gives at least some result. But that doesn't mean you know what you are doing. That's exactly the danger of genetic research. These researchers are messing with the basics of life without knowing what they are doing. This can only end in a complete disaster. GMO foods are known to cause cancer and other diseases at the short term. But what will these crops do at the longer term? Nobody has any idea, but it won't be anything good.
And doctors are now trying to replace "faulty genes" in embryos, to get a healthy baby. I don't know if they have already succeeded with that, but this kind of messing with genes can only end up in a gigantic disaster. If a baby with replaced genes will be born, what does that mean? Will it die soon, or will it get sick soon, or will it be infertile? Maybe the baby won't get sick and will the disaster first

happen in the next generation, or the generation after that. Maybe something else will happen. We don't know and it's absolutely impossible to predict. We can only observe the disaster when it happens.

Geneticists play god and history has shown that this always ends up in disasters. Reality is that genes are way too complicated for our human brains and we will never understand it. Forget it. We will never get any further than wild assumptions and dangerous theories. We all need to get rid of the obsession that genes cause all kinds of things. Most probably they don't and if they have something to do with diseases then this will be in an extremely complicated way.

Useless and harmful

Many decades of genetic research has brought us nothing good. It has mainly brought us a lot of unnecessary medical treatments, which just harm. It has told people that they cannot do anything to influence their own health, making them victims of their genes. Genetic research hasn't brought us cures for diseases and it doesn't do anything to prevent diseases. It has resulted in a lot of highly questionable practices, which for many people are ethically unacceptable. Abortions because a baby has a certain gene are already quite common. Embryo selection for genes has not proven either to do any good. And soon people with a "genetic disease" will be told not to get children. What will happen in the future is something nobody knows, but if we keep obsessed with genes nothing good will come from it.

Genetics is for at least 99.9% "must be" science.

3. Viruses and bacteria

Viruses are funny things with an undeserved bad reputation. They got that bad reputation when at the point of discovery everything went wrong.

Some time ago I felt like there was something not right with the theory of viruses, so I started to investigate. And very quickly I found out that the whole of virology was based on nothing but assumptions. You can do a bit of investigation yourself and find the same things. Any book or video about virology will tell you how things happened. Someone had a sick plant and the scientists couldn't find bacteria or fungi that could be the cause. They started to look for something and after a lot of processing, filtering and studying they found something they called a virus. (I'm not sure what they found exactly, as the electron microscope wasn't invented till 1931). And they blindly concluded that they had found a new micro-organism and that this micro-organism was the cause of the disease. This wasn't based on anything, but the idea stuck. The only correct conclusion would have been that there was a virus in a sick plant. The disease could also have caused the virus, or the two could have been completely unrelated. But virology (and largely also bacteriology) are in the category "if the only tool you have is a hammer then the whole world will look like a nail". If the only tool you have to explain disease is micro-organisms, then that's all you will see. It doesn't mean that your explanations are correct. (It appeared later that the plant they used had a nutrient deficiency. Multiple of deficiency diseases have been attributed to viruses since.)

What is a virus?
So what exactly are viruses? That's a really good question and there aren't a lot of answers. At least no answers that make sense and are based on scientific evidence. The problem is the size of the virus. Viruses are extremely small, way too small to be seen under a standard light microscope. And electron microscopes are so powerful that they shoot the viruses into pieces. No virologist has ever seen a complete virus, let alone a live virus. Let that sink in for a moment. If these scientists can't see a live virus, then how do they know that the virus causes disease? And how it causes disease? And how it spreads? The truth is that they don't know these things. They

assume them and if they don't even have enough information to make an assumption they just fabricate something. Once you start digging into virology you will find nothing but wild assumptions and a lot of fantasy.

So what are the scientists talking about when they say they have discovered a new virus? They are talking about tiny pieces of DNA they have found under the electron microscope. They take all these pieces and puzzle them together till they have what they assume is a full genome. Then they assume that this genome is the virus they are looking for. And then they assume that this virus is the cause of a certain disease. And then they tell the whole world that they have discovered the cause of the disease and from there the story takes off. But it was never more than a story.

So if nobody can see a complete virus, then what about all those pictures of viruses? If you do an Internet search you will get truckloads of pictures of flu viruses, measles viruses, AIDS viruses and all kinds of other viruses. They are round or square, with spots or lines, with knobs or spikes and they come in a variety of colours. But take a closer look at these photos and compare multiple pictures of the same virus. And then you will see the differences. One and the same virus can have big knobs or small knobs, spots or no spots, a thick membrane or a thin one and they come in a variety of colours. Usually (but not always) different pictures of the same virus show some similarities, but that's about it. These are not photos of viruses. They are nice artwork and nothing more than that. But let's be honest: they look attractive and scientific enough to fool most people. (Electron microscopes only give black-and-white pictures. Colours are added to make them look more convincing.)

Dead material
There is no consensus whether viruses are dead or alive, though most scientists nowadays agree that they are dead.[4] The theory is that a virus is nothing more than a package of DNA and protein, that cannot live on its own. It needs a host to reproduce. That immediately causes a big problem, for how does a dead substance enter a host? And how does it come to life? It must become alive to

---

[4] In a desperate attempt to make reality fit their theories there are also scientists who say that viruses are "semi-alive". What that means is a mystery.

reproduce, but something dead cannot come to life. So far I haven't read any kind of explanation for this problem. When things don't add up scientists usually simply ignore it.

This also creates a problem with the theory of mutations. Viruses are said to mutate and therefore cause disease again in people who should have immunity from a previous infection. This only happens in viruses that meet the socio-political criteria. People get the flu every year, so the virus must be able to mutate. The measles virus must be stable, for else people would also get it every year and they don't. (Here you notice again that medical science is riddled with "must be's.") But how does dead material mutate?

Another problem is how viruses spread. They are said to jump from host to host and that way they keep themselves going. The vaccination theory of herd immunity is based on the idea that if nobody gets the disease there won't be a host left and the virus will disappear. The problem is that this theory has been proven wrong again and again. When there is an outbreak of disease, e.g. measles, then the outbreak had to start somewhere. How did this patient zero get the virus? This has become a problem, so out of necessity governments and doctors came with the statements that the person "has imported it", usually from overseas. This usually doesn't make any sense, but it's the only explanation that's left. There have been cases of children with measles and chickenpox at Australian cattle stations. These kids hadn't had contact with the outside world for months, so where did they get the virus? These viruses are supposed to have incubation periods of just a few days.

Incubation period
That brings us to the problem of the incubation period. This is one of those things that are in complete conflict with the theory of viruses. If a virus causes a disease it should do so in a short period of time, not more than a few hours. If you have a strong immune system this will attack the virus at entrance and you won't get sick. There is no room in the theory for any kind of incubation period. The incubation period is based on a social necessity. Children got measles or mumps when they hadn't been in contact with other kids for days, so the infection "must have happened" before that. And so there "must be" an incubation period. As there are usually loads of people with the flu the incubation period for the flu is very short. With childhood

diseases this varies from a few days to a week. But with a disease like hepatitis B this incubation period is said to be some 30 years. In 30 years the body hasn't attacked and removed the virus and it hasn't gotten sick. That makes for a very strange virus. Why on earth would the virus wait that long with making someone sick? It has no use for waiting that long. And why can't the body remove it? What's so special about this virus? Nobody has ever answered those questions. They can't answer them, for it doesn't make any sense whatsoever. The same story goes for shingles, which is said to be a "dormant virus" after you have gotten the chickenpox. Again, why doesn't the immune system remove the virus completely? What's so different about this virus? Most people who get shingles only get is once. So does that mean that after that the immune system has finally eliminated it? Shingles usually happens in older people. Why does the virus take so long to resurface?

The last few years the World Health Organisation together with the mainstream media have created one viral scare after another. We have had the swine flu and the bird flu, SARS and MERS, Ebola and chikungunya. And the last one was the Zika hype. This one is actually quite interesting. In January 2016 hardly anyone had heard about Zika, but as soon as the media scare started test kits were available all over the world, in all hospitals and laboratories. That makes you wonder what they are actually testing for. And in media reports scientists admitted that they actually know very little about the virus, but a few months later they knew at once what kind of diseases the virus causes and how it spreads. If anything belongs in the mythology books it's the Zika virus, together with all the other "hype viruses". These viruses are adjusted according to the political needs. There is no science behind it.

At the same time there are many people who say that these viruses are man-made with the intention to destroy the world. But as I explained above, viruses don't cause disease and are nothing more than some DNA. Nobody has any idea what a virus is, let alone that they could design one in a lab that would cause a disease that spreads in a certain way. Man-made viruses belong in scary science fiction movies, but have nothing to do with reality.

Bacteria
So you know now that you don't need to worry about viruses. But

what about bacteria? Bacteria have been known for longer than viruses, because they are much bigger and you can easily see them under a light microscope. They are a completely different kind of micro-organism than viruses. They can replicate on their own and they are absolutely connected to disease.

Bacteria are the most important organisms on earth, as they are the cleaners. They make organic waste fall apart, so that it can be used again by plants and trees in an everlasting cycle. We also have loads of bacteria in and on our body and we should be happy with that. Without those bacteria we would be dead very quickly.

It looks like bacteria can cause disease. Infected wounds are really bad and food poisoning can make you very sick. On the other hand we have bacteria in our gut that digest our food and make sure we can use all the nutrients in it. That's the reason why people have started to talk about "good" and "bad" bacteria. But that's not correct. There are no bad bacteria. All bacteria are necessary. But you can have good bacteria at the wrong place. E. coli bacteria are very important in your bowel, but can be nasty if ingested.

Not the enemy

The different faces of bacteria make them very interesting, but unfortunately the medical profession doesn't see that bacteria are really important. They see that people can get sick from them and that makes them all bad. Kill them with antibiotics, as they are your enemies. But they are not. It's always said that antibiotics have saved millions of lives and on the surface that looks correct. But this is not necessarily so. Antibiotics kill all the bacteria that show up in case of disease and at the same time kill an awful lot of bacteria in your gut, that you need so badly to stay healthy. The latter is acknowledged as a problem, but the first is seen as a great idea. But it's not.

The bacteria that cause tuberculosis, whooping cough or meningitis (just to name a few diseases) are not bad ones. Many people carry these bacteria without getting sick. And if you assume that nothing in nature is coincidence and that everything has a place, then those bacteria are there for a reason. Even if you don't know what that reason is.

So just killing all bacteria is not a great idea. Antibiotics are also highly toxic. So could it be that in killing our friends in large numbers has actually taken more lives than it saved? I would say that that's a likely possibility. On the other hand, natural antibiotics have been known for a long time and have none of these issues. Nature knows exactly how to handle things, but doctors wanted to know better and it has caused loads and loads of problems.

Immunity

So what about immunity against infectious diseases? To answer any question about immunity we first need to deal with the concept of infectious diseases. This idea is as old as the human race. Diseases showed up in clusters and it's not hard to see how people concluded that one person must infect the other. But this has no scientific basis at all. This is hard to accept, as the idea of diseases being contagious is something we have all grown up with. But reality has shown otherwise. I strongly recommend the book "Bechamp or Pasteur?"[5] In chapter 1 you can read a report from Florence Nightingale.

> *"I was brought up to believe that smallpox, for instance, was a thing of which there was once a first specimen in the world, which went on propagating itself, in a perpetual chain of descent, just as there was a first dog (or a first pair of dogs), and that smallpox would not begin itself, any more than a new dog would begin without there having been a parent dog.*
>
> *Since then I have seen with my own eyes and smelled with my own nose smallpox growing up in first specimens, either in closed rooms or in overcrowded wards, where it could not by any possibility have been 'caught', but must have begun.*
>
> *I have seen diseases begin, grow up, and turn into one another. Now dogs do not turn into cats.*
> *I have seen, for instance, with a little overcrowding, continued fever grow up; and with a little more, typhoid fever; and with a little more, typhus, and all in the same ward or hut."*

---

[5] Bechamp or Pasteur? by Ethel D. Hume. Generally for sale as hard copy, or a free digital download at http://www.mnwelldir.org/docs/history/biographies/Bechamp-or-Pasteur.pdf

Wherever the diseases come from, not from someone who infects other people. They come from inside us, not from an outside source.

So what about immunity? There are two different interpretations of the word immunity. The first one is the concept that once you have had a certain disease you will never get it again. The second one is the situation that your body is strong enough to handle whatever happens in the environment.

The first use of the word immunity is very generally accepted, but that doesn't make it true. You can easily find out yourself that this isn't correct. Just ask around if people have had diseases like chickenpox, measles or whooping cough more than once and you will be surprised how many people had such diseases multiple times. It's not a rare exception, but actually it's quite common. You can only conclude that getting these diseases does not mean you have life-long protection. This whole idea is based on folklore. It was noticed that many people get certain diseases only once and it's not hard to see how "many" became "everyone". And once such an idea has become generally accepted nobody notices anymore all those cases where the theory proves incorrect. There simply is not something like life-long immunity against infectious diseases.

So what about the second type of immunity? The idea is that "germ + immune system = disease or not disease". If you have a strong immune system you won't get sick. But also this proves wrong every time. No matter how healthy children are, they often get measles and chickenpox anyway. On the other hand, healthy children get through these diseases without any problems, where sick, weak and malnourished children can die from them.

But imagine that this theory would be true. When your immune system is weakened by hunger or stress then you would get a viral or bacterial disease a lot easier. The world is full of viruses and bacteria, which means that if you would be weak enough to catch one you would catch them all. The human species wouldn't survive very long, as we all have times that our bodies are weakened.

In my book "The Fiction Of Science" I write about the soldiers in the American civil war.

"During the American Civil War the soldiers were tired, stressed, lonely and malnourished. Many of them got so badly injured that arms and legs had to be amputated. These amputations weren't done in a proper operating theatre. They were done on tables in field tents, often in the rain and mud. Nobody washed their hands and antibiotics weren't available. Under these circumstances you wouldn't expect a lot of soldiers to survive, but the remarkable fact is that the vast majority did not develop gangrene and their wounds healed without infection."[6]

No more proof is needed that the theory of immune systems is simply not true. In reality nobody has ever found where in our body the immune system is positioned. A variety of theories go around, which have made it into the mainstream medical mythology. But there is no scientific basis for these theories. The problem is that immunologists assume that there is an immune system and from there they started searching for things that proved their assumption correct. But when the basic assumption is incorrect, then everything else will also be wrong.

What then?
So what determines whether we get sick or not, whether we survive a disease or not? I'm not sure if this question already has an answer. Nobody has looked for it, as they are way too busy identifying an immune system that doesn't exist. So researchers don't look for other options. But there are observations. People who have good food and clean water have a much bigger chance not to get sick or to easily survive a disease. And happiness and lack of stress also greatly contribute to health.
On the other hand the above-mentioned story of the American soldiers proves that this is not the case in every situation.

There is just one conclusion that is very obvious: whatever theories go around about viruses and bacteria are wrong. They all belong in the book of medical mythology.

---

[6] The Fiction Of Science, chapter 1: germs

4. Vaccinations

In a book about medical mythology you can't go around vaccinations. Not only are they entirely myth based, but they are also the backbone of the medical system. If you would take vaccines away the whole system would start to crumble.

Many books have been written about the topic and most of them focus on the dangers of vaccinations.[7] And the vast majority of people who do not accept vaccines do so because "the dangers outweigh the benefits". But this is not true. Vaccines don't have any benefits, which leaves only the dangers. But the idea that vaccines have at least some effect is deeply rooted in society. So let's have a look at the diseases that have a vaccine.

Smallpox
The whole vaccination scheme started with the smallpox vaccine. Edward Jenner used pus from cowpox to protect people against smallpox. This didn't work, because it simply could not work. The idea that infection with cowpox would protect against smallpox was common folklore in the 1700's in England. But what exactly was cowpox?
Cowpox was a disease of the udders of milk cows. Bulls were not affected and neither was beef cattle. Calves that weren't milked yet didn't get the disease. And the cowpox never got any further than the udders. It's not so hard to see that the cowpox was a disease that was spread by milkmaids. And that it had absolutely nothing to do with the smallpox. There are different theories about what the cowpox were exactly, but that is not even relevant. What is relevant is that the vaccine could not have worked. After the cowpox Jenner still used horses, rabbits and other animals that had some kind of skin disease and it's not hard to believe that his dirty cocktails caused a variety of infections in this patients.

Smallpox was a skin disease and most skin diseases are just a way of the body to get rid of toxic substances. As the smallpox vaccine was a remarkably dirty concoction it's not so strange that smallpox was more common in the vaccinated than in the unvaccinated.

---

[7] Books I recommend are "Vaccine-nation" by Andreas Moritz, "VACCeptable injuries" by Markus Heinze and "Vaccine epidemic" by Louise Habakus and Mary Holland.

Polio

But what about polio? Didn't polio disappear after the vaccine was introduced? The polio vaccine was the moment that virology really took off. Till then it had been a not very well known science, but this would change dramatically. So what was polio?

The first outbreaks of polio happened in the USA, shortly after a new pesticide had been introduced. Groups of paralysed children were found in the apple orchards. Apples have always needed large amounts of pesticides and the lead and arsenic caused serious neurological damage to the children (adults were not as badly affected though they didn't always completely escape). Wherever this new pesticide was introduced polio would follow immediately. It was impossible not to see the connection, but for economical reasons it was ignored. When the first poison was banned it was replaced with another and another and eventually with DDT. And polio outbreaks kept happening everywhere. There were more interesting things about polio, which clearly showed that it was not an infectious disease. Infectious diseases were always worse in winter, when low temperatures, lack of sunshine and poor quality food would weaken the people. These diseases also always have been worse among the poor. But not so with polio.

Polio outbreaks only happened in summer, starting soon after the spraying of crops started. And it mainly effected children from wealthier families. The very poor usually escaped. These are huge red flags, which were routinely ignored. DDT was sprayed generously on everything and everyone. Because polio was thought to be spread by mosquitoes houses were sprayed with large amounts of DDT. But only by those who could afford it. The poor would swat the mosquitoes with a newspaper. The rich could also afford more fruit, with large amounts of pesticides. Again, it's not so hard to see what was the cause of polio.

But banning the pesticides didn't seem to be an option. Looking for a virus on the other hand seemed really scientific. But it wasn't. The researchers simply started to look for a virus that met their criteria. And there are an unlimited number of viruses, so if you search long enough you will find one that can be used. So they took an innocent bowel virus and blamed it for polio. But reality is that the "polio virus" never was even related to polio, let alone that it caused it.

Even if you believe that viruses cause disease, then still it's obvious that the polio virus cannot cause polio. That makes the polio virus not a myth, but a hoax.

So what about the disappearance of polio? Also that is a hoax. Once DDT got banned polio stopped showing up in outbreaks, but it never disappeared. It was simply renamed. There is a long list of diagnoses that in 1950 simply would have been labelled "polio". This goes from aseptic meningitis and Guillain Barre syndrome to multiple sclerosis and muscular dystrophy. Reality is that nowadays there are more people with paralytic diseases and more people on ventilators than there ever were before the polio vaccine was introduced.

Hepatitis

Hepatitis comes with a number of letters, from A to E, though more letters are coming. It refers to liver inflammation and is attributed to different viruses, though at the same time they are the same viruses. When you dig into hepatitis the theories don't remotely add up and are basically all over the place.

The hepatitis B vaccine is generally given to babies. So what is this disease said to be? It's said that it's caused by a virus, which is transferred by blood contact or sex, so therefore it's mainly a disease from IV drug users and prostitutes. This has never been proven, but that doesn't stop anyone. These two groups have a variety of other things in common that could cause disease, but they are routinely ignored in favour of a virus.

The hepatitis B virus is said to infect a person and then stay dormant for 20-40 years. And then it can cause liver damage. Why would the virus stay dormant for that long? Can't the liver damage be caused by something else? With so many years in between that's extremely likely.

When you start searching in the PubMed database you will soon find that selenium supplements take away the symptoms of hepatitis B (and all other types as well, but the hepatitis B vaccine is the only one that's routinely given at the moment.) The explanation is that selenium suppresses the virus, but a much more logical explanation is of course that hepatitis is simply a selenium deficiency disease. IV drug users and prostitutes usually have very poor eating habits and will likely suffer from chronic lack of selenium (and other nutrients).

If they change their lifestyles and start eating normally again the "virus disappears". And yes, hepatitis B is also common in the general population in certain areas in the world. And they happen to be areas with low selenium in the soil.

The medical profession has a history of attributing nutrient deficiency diseases to viruses, with beriberi and pellagra as two infamous examples. Hepatitis is just another one.

Measles, mumps, rubella and chickenpox

These are common childhood diseases, which of course are attributed to viruses. But nobody can explain why these viruses usually only infect children of a certain age. Well, that's how it used to be, but the last ten years or so there are more and more stories of these diseases showing up out of the normal age range.

The symptoms of these diseases point into the direction of a clean-up, though likely other things are involved too. That could be the reason why some children get these diseases multiple times and others not at all. The more rubbish piles up in the body, the bigger the need for a clean-up. I have tried to figure out if these diseases already existed 500 years ago, but that's simply not possible as nobody kept records. There are some medical records, but they require interpretation and that can't be reliable. Considering how much toxic stuff the world puts into our bodies nowadays it's likely that these are new diseases.

It's known that breastfeeding usually keeps these childhood diseases away till the child is older. That could be because breast milk is a miracle fluid that we know very little about. It could also be that commercial baby formulas add to the load on the baby's body and soon a clean-up is necessary. And if teenagers or young adults get the childhood diseases, could it be that they simply get it for the second or third time? Because everyone believes that you cannot get these diseases multiple times it's very well possible that the mild case in childhood is forgotten. These are just theories, but they make a lot more sense than a virus that jumps up out of nowhere to make adults sick with childhood diseases.

The mumps vaccine was never invented because the mumps is a dangerous disease. It was always an "economic vaccine": if your child doesn't get sick, you don't need to take time off work. It is only quite recently that the myth has shown up that mumps is dangerous for boys, as it makes them sterile. Reality is that sterility because of mumps is so rare that no country has even statistics about it. In post-pubescent males mumps can cause inflammation of the testis, which occasionally can cause sterility. But this inflammation is almost always one-sided and if sterility happens in one testis then the other one can still produce enough sperm to populate the world. Double-sided inflammation is rare and as the single-sided sterility is already pretty uncommon you can see how remote the chances are. It's not an issue.

And then rubella, which is said to be dangerous during pregnancy. A few decades ago rubella during pregnancy was said to cause eye problems in the baby. But somehow a long list of problems is now attributed to rubella and it has been named "congenital rubella syndrome". (Keep in mind that the word "syndrome" usually means that doctors don't have any idea what they are talking about.) And quite recently chickenpox has also been added as dangerous during pregnancy, but that fear hasn't spread widely yet. That is simply because the vaccine isn't available in most countries yet, so there's no point in scaring people.

So what's the truth about this syndrome? It's completely based on folklore. There is no science behind it and there's no proof that rubella is risky for an unborn baby. The whole theory is based on observations and the wish for an explanation. When a baby is born with any kind of congenital defect parents want to know why this happened. And so doctors start searching for explanations. And if you search long enough you can find something. A few blind babies after pregnancy rubella was probably enough to start the myth. But let's do some simple math. A certain number of babies is born with a congenital disorder. A certain number of women will get rubella during pregnancy. That means that by chance alone some women will get a handicapped baby after they had rubella. But most women who get a handicapped baby did not have rubella during pregnancy. And most women who did have rubella deliver a healthy baby. The numbers are all over the place and there is simply no correlation. We can send this one straight to the medical mythology.

Tetanus

The fear for tetanus is getting hammered into us and doctors routinely give the vaccines to about anyone and everyone who comes in with some kind of injury. But what exactly is tetanus? Generally tetanus is ascribed to a bacteria that lives in manure and sometimes in the soil. It's an anaerobe bacteria (it lives without oxygen and dies in the presence of oxygen) and you would need a deep puncture wound from an infected object to be infected with the bacteria. But an infection doesn't mean tetanus. It's very likely that many people get infected with these bacteria without ever getting sick. But that's not all. There are also plenty of cases of people with tetanus who did not have an infection with the bacteria and often never even had a deep puncture would from a possibly infected object.

So what does that mean? If you add these two up you can only come to the conclusion that tetanus and the "tetanus bacteria" have such a lose correlation that it's just another germ that is blamed for a disease that it has nothing to do with. Probably many people have this bacteria in their body and it doesn't cause disease. When someone gets tetanus and the bacteria are found the poor bacteria get blamed when they were there already for decades and never caused any harm. This kind of medical mythology is common, as doctors so badly want to blame germs for everything and anything. So they search for a germ and find one and without any proof this wild assumption becomes fact. But the researchers routinely ignore everything that goes against their theory, creating one myth after another.

Diphtheria, whooping cough and tuberculosis

I put these three together, as they are all diseases of the respiratory system. And they are all ascribed to bacteria. But there is a problem here. Many people carry these bacteria in their throats and lungs without getting sick. Obviously the bacteria need to be there and are not harmful. But now there is another question: how many people get these diseases without testing positive for the bacteria? That question doesn't have an answer, because doctors are so stuck in their medical paradigms that they won't give a diagnosis of any of these diseases if the patient doesn't test positive. If someone has all the symptoms of whooping cough, but a negative test, then the doctor will diagnose anything but whooping cough.

But we know that many people get tetanus without the bacteria. So it's likely that many people get whooping cough or diphtheria without the bacteria. (Why do we know this about tetanus and not about whooping cough, tuberculosis or diphtheria? I can't answer that question with certainty, but it might be that tetanus is simply harder to diagnose as something else, as the symptoms are quite unusual. Lung diseases are more common and an alternative diagnosis isn't so hard to find.)

Meningitis, HiB and pneumonia
Three more diseases that are ascribed to bacteria. They are serious and people can die from them. But also with these it's a known fact that many people carry the bacteria without getting sick. It's not the bacteria that cause the disease. They just show up as a result of disease.

Because doctors don't know the nature of bacteria they usually treat these diseases with high doses of antibiotics and yes, the bacteria go then. But the reason why they were there isn't solved and so the patient is set up for a lot of other problems. On top of that antibiotics also kill the good bacteria and that weakens the patient, especially if it's a little kid. The result of that can be disastrous.

If there is a need to act quickly then natural antibiotics are a good medicine. They do solve the infection, likely without killing all the bacteria at once. And they leave the gut bacteria alone. Natural therapies respect bacteria instead of killing them like they are the worst enemy.

Rotavirus
I have already explained that viruses don't cause disease, so the name "rotavirus" is a weird one. The disease is heavy diarrhoea and the main risk is dehydration. If this is dealt with properly it's just unpleasant, but not dangerous. Exclusive breastfeeding prevents this disease. Considering that diarrhoea is a way of the body to get rid of unwanted stuff I wonder if this disease isn't really prevented by breastfeeding, but is actually caused by formula. It is a pretty recent phenomenon and new diseases don't just happen. They are caused by something in the environment. Looking at commercial baby formula makes sense, but nobody has ever done that of course. Baby formula is way too profitable to get any kind of bad publicity.

Influenza

This used to be a pretty bad disease, but it has become milder and milder the last ten years. That's not because the disease itself has changed, but because everything and anything that makes people sick in winter is now categorised as the flu.

So what about the flu virus? Once you dig into it the theory of the flu virus is actually quite hilarious. There are a gazillion of flu particles, but nevertheless only one of them mutates and that happens in Asia (why in Asia?) Researchers can find that one mutation to make the flu shot (good luck searching for a virus on a large continent). Then the virus starts multiplying. It can only do that in a host, but somehow nobody gets sick with this mutated virus. Then the virus starts to travel around the world, again without making anyone sick. It first goes to the Northern Hemisphere and six months later it travels to the Southern Hemisphere (how does the virus know where to go?) It travels by plane, boat, train, bus, car and carriage to every little corner of the world (without making anyone sick) and then… it waits. It waits till winter starts (whenever that might be in all the different countries) and then at once it starts to make everyone sick. And once winter is over it disappears, till it mutates again and the whole story starts from the beginning.

It's obvious that this story is void of any kind of science. It goes against all other theories about viruses as well. This is not even medical mythology. It's a fabricated absurdity, meant to sell flu shots. This deserves a place in the Museum of Absurdities, not in a medical practice.

Spanish flu

In any discussion about vaccines not only the smallpox and polio are brought into the discussion, but also the Spanish flu will show up. That was terrible and highly contagious, wasn't it? Well, it sure was terrible, but it wasn't Spanish and it wasn't flu. This drama was entirely caused by vaccinations themselves.

In the early 1900's there was a lot of experimenting with the production of vaccines and the shots were all kinds of things, against all kinds of diseases. Modern vaccines are highly dirty concoctions, but the ones made in this period were even worse. European soldiers that were sent to war were injected with these vaccines and many never made it to the battle field, because they died or got very sick from the vaccines. Then a problem arose for the manufacturers (and the governments that paid for the vaccines). The war was over a lot earlier than had been expected and there were loads of vaccine doses left, that would soon expire. So they were distributed among the ordinary people. The story was launched that all these soldiers would come home with all these dreadful diseases and everyone had to get vaccinated against them. The result was that millions of people got very sick and died. To hide the origins the myth of the Spanish flu was spread.

Those who got vaccinated got sick, but those who didn't get vaccinated never got the dreaded disease. Countries that completely refused the vaccines never got one case of the disease.

Not that much has changed since. There are still loads of diseases that are caused by vaccines and scientists are quick to find a germ that can be blamed for them. And then vaccines are made against these germs, causing more vaccine induced diseases. The only difference is that nobody got the idea to make a vaccine against Spanish flu.

Conclusion
Though the diseases that have vaccines can be nasty, none of them is caused by the germs that are blamed for them. Therefore no vaccine can have any preventative effect whatsoever. They are a hoax. They come with a lot of danger and no benefits. The choice should be a no-brainer.

5. Drugs

It's not possible to write a book about the medical system without mentioning drugs. The conventional medical system is entirely based on pharmaceuticals. Without pharmaceuticals doctors wouldn't know what to do, as they have little else. They can send a patient to a physiotherapist or a psychologist, but in most cases they print a script. If something is that popular it must be safe and highly effective, you would think. And most people think that drugs are well researched and wouldn't be on the market if they wouldn't be safe. Ask any doctor and they will tell you that drugs are very well researched and that it's hard to get them approved, so they are great things. And they will have to believe that, because if they would admit to the truth they couldn't do their work anymore. But it's one big myth, and a very dangerous one.

History

Pharmaceuticals are a quite new thing. In the mid 1800's it slowly started to become a business with substances like morphine and aspirin. But it was first in the 1900's that this industry really took off. For a big part his was because in the USA pharmaceutical businesses managed to take over universities. Within a few decades medical students mainly learnt about how to treat diseases with drugs and other options like herbs or homeopathic remedies were pushed to the fringe. Other countries followed quickly and 100 years later we are stuck with a pharmaceuticals based medical system and everything else is "alternative", though many of these have existed for thousands of years.

Once the pharmaceutical industry had managed to take over the medical system the number of drugs exploded. There is a lot of money in drugs and when one company has invented a successful drug others want to get their piece of the cake. But drugs have patents and so other manufacturers need to find a way around that. They change a tiny bit of the profitable substance, so that it still has pretty much the same effect. And then they push it on the people. You can imagine that this creates competition and the number of patients with a disease is limited. In all other industries competition means better quality and lower prices, but not with pharmaceuticals. For this is a very strange category. The person who will take it is not the person who decides that it's necessary and in most cases it's a third party (the insurance company or the government) that pays for it. The doctor doesn't care about the price and the insurance company doesn't care about the quality. And the patient doesn't have a choice for another product.

Research

It's a very stubborn myth that pharmaceutical drugs are well researched. Everyone wants to believe that, because else you would feel pretty stupid taking a drug that has never been proven to be useful. But when you take a look into the process you are in for a shock. When a company has developed a new substance this will first be tested on animals. If the animals survive it the next step will be to test it on a group of healthy humans. These people get quite well paid for this, for else nobody would risk their health. In this stage the fraud already sets in. For if the substance has shown to be financially promising, then safety takes the backseat. It is not unusual that in this first test stage loads of nasty problems show up, which are then swept under the carpet. Manipulating study results is really not that hard and outright fraud is actually a common practice. You just don't mention that someone got a heart attack, or kidney failure, or attempted suicide. These people just dropped out of the trial and are simply not counted. And if the problems are too big, the company simply stops the trial. They have no obligation whatsoever to publish the results of every trial they do for a drug. Only completed trials are used. So if it appears that things go wrong, then they stop the trial halfway and start a new one, with a new design.

The groups of test people are not randomly chosen either. Usually young, healthy people are used, but once a drug gets approved it will be prescribed to sick and older people. You can expect this to go wrong.

If in phase 2 things are not too bad then phase 3 trials start. This means that the drug will be given to people who have the disease the drug needs to treat. This is done with a randomised, double blind, placebo controlled trial. One group gets the drug and the other group gets a fake pill and nobody knows what they get. That way the effect of taking a pill should be removed. It sounds so scientific, but it's not. Drugs have unwanted effects, usually called side effects, though this is a misleading term. People who participate in these trials are usually familiar with the kind of side effects they can expect. So when they notice e.g. a dry mouth, some nausea, dizziness or an itchy skin, they know they are in the drug group. This means that usually within a couple of days the double-blind part of the trial is already over. Those who take the drug know they take it and as these people have pretty high expectations of the new drug they will likely improve. This is not just a strong placebo effect. Measuring the effect of a drug is not just a matter of lab tests and scans. It's for a big part the patient reporting how they feel. And if you expect to feel better you will write down that there is an improvement, even if there is none. This goes especially for psychiatric drugs, when tests are completely unavailable. The efficacy of those drugs comes entirely from what the patients tell. It's completely meaningless, but nevertheless this is standard practice and most people think that these "randomised" trials are very important and give very good, objective information.

Another problem with these kind of trials is that there is no definition of a placebo. It must be an inactive substance, but this is not further defined. But let's say that you test a new diabetes drug and the placebo is a sugar pill, then those on the placebo are likely to do worse than those on the drug. Or reversed: the drug is effective. The placebo can be anything that is likely to have a bad effect on the patients involved in the test.

But at least large numbers of patients are involved in these trials, right? Unfortunately this is another myth. It looks like it, for pharmaceutical businesses are masters in manipulating numbers. For the ordinary person it's almost impossible to figure out how many people were involved in the beginning, in the end, in which study and how many dropped out early or later. If a study has been published as involving 10,000 people it's not uncommon that the number was actually 400.

Effects

So when a drug has been shown to be effective, what is it effective with? The patients assume that a drug will make them feel better or make them live longer, but this is rarely the case. Take popular diabetes drugs. They are designed to lower blood sugar and they do that pretty well. This might make the patient feel better, though type 2 diabetes often goes unnoticed, so the effect of the drug will likely also go unnoticed. The only way the patients know the drug is working is by getting a blood glucose test done. So are these drugs good for the health of the patient? No, they aren't. For though the sugar is down, the insulin remains high and it's the high insulin that will cause the damage. Still the drugs are marketed as highly effective. This is called a "surrogate endpoint". If the drug is effective for this endpoint it can get easily approved. But the patients don't care much about the surrogate. They want to be healthier and live longer. Another example of such a surrogate endpoint is cholesterol and the statin medications that lower this. Those drugs are pretty good in lowering cholesterol. But they do not lower death rates. On the contrary, they increase death rates. But the manufacturers don't tell that to the doctors and so the patients don't know. It's an absurd system, where the industry can invent its own theories and as long as the product meets the theories that's good enough. And what happens when ten years later it appears that surrogate endpoint was a fantasy and that drugs don't do any good? Well, diabetes medication, statins and blood pressure lowering drugs (just to name a few common ones) are still on the market, though they have been proven to be dangerous and useless. Once doctors have started to prescribe drugs they are not keen to stop with it. For then they have to admit that they were fooled and doctors don't like to do that.

Approval process

So phase 3 trials are over and the results are positive enough to approach the different government agencies to search for approval. Every country has a different process for this, but in the end they are largely the same. Every country likes to believe that their system is much better and that bad drugs really won't get approved. That only happens in other countries. Forget it. It's hard to predict what drug will get approved in what country. A drug might be popular in the

USA and not even approved in France. Another drug might be approved quickly in Belgium, but never makes it to the market in Australia and the USA. It seems pretty random. Nevertheless it helps a lot if a drug gets approved in a few important countries. Other countries are more likely to approve it too. The approval process can be lengthy, but the industry has ways to speed this up. A common way is to involve doctors in the country in "research". They are asked to give the so far unapproved drug to their patients, for a sum of money and for their name in the research reports. Many doctors fall for that and they start handing out the new drug. And once they are in the habit they are likely to put pressure on the government authority to approve the drug, which "is so great" and "my patients shouldn't be denied it". The pharmaceutical industry are masters in manipulation and any doctor who talks to a representative will fall for it. It's almost impossible not to get influenced.

So what happens if the drug gets approved? Then the marketing starts. Actually, marketing often already starts before a drug is approved, to warm doctors and public to the new drug. As soon as the drug is available in pharmacies aggressive advertising starts and doctors get visits from pharmaceutical representatives. Loads of visits, for it takes time to convince a doctor to prescribe this new drug. That usually doesn't happen in a few days. Only in the USA and New Zealand it's allowed to advertise prescription medications directly to the public. But the industry has found ways around that. In all other countries they advertise the disease and they do it in such a way that whoever feels sick will be very happy to take the new pill. For of course at the moment the disease advertising starts the doctors are bombarded with information about this new drug that is so good. Patients will ask for the drug and the doctor will prescribe. Mission accomplished.

After the approval
So what happens then? Now phase 4 of the research stars. This is called "post marketing surveillance". As I described the pre-approval research usually involves only small groups of people, who take the drug for a short period of time. People often think that such trials take a year or longer, but they never do. The trial usually takes a few weeks, but rarely more than three months. So if 1000 people take a

drug for three weeks it's unlikely that a lot of problems will show up. But when the drug gets generally prescribed and a million people take it for a year or longer (which is very common nowadays) then all the problems will start to emerge. While doctors like to believe that new drugs have been proven to be safe, reality shows that around 50% of the drugs that were approved as safe have very dangerous side-effects. Most of them are taken off the market within five years. How it's possible that some stay on the market is something I can't explain.

But no matter how dangerous, some drugs remain popular for a long time. These are the "blockbuster" drugs, which make the manufacturers a lot of money. $1 billion a year profit is not unusual. This is mainly achieved because the drugs have a patent. How long a patent lasts depends on different factors, but after 20 years it's over. And then the price drops a lot, as everyone can make it and doctors are nowadays quite happy to prescribe the generic product. But there are ways around this. A popular one is to get the drug approved for a different condition. Drugs have wanted and unwanted effects. The unwanted effects are called side effects, but they are just effects. It can happen that a side effect is not just nasty, but an interesting option for more profit. When a drug to lower blood pressure causes sleepiness, then it's a good idea to sell the same drug (but with a different name!) as a sleeping pill, with side effect "can lower the blood pressure". And the new drug has a new patent and the money keeps flowing.

Another way to deal with it is to make a tiny change to your substance. As I mentioned above the competition often has already done this, but there are always other options. And when you have a new substance you can sell it as a new drug in the same category, but that might not be the best way to go. The market is full, so it's better to see if you can sell your new pill for a completely new disease. A popular (but very dangerous) anti-depressant drug lost its patent a while ago. Not long after almost the same substance, from the same manufacturer came on the market as an ADHD drug. But this time it was marketed to children, a group that "doesn't take enough drugs yet". The dangers of the drug are the same, but now you get 8 years old children who are suicidal or homicidal.[8] But somehow the drugs get approved and the doctors prescribe them.

So why is almost everyone taking the drugs that the doctors prescribe? And why do so many people keep taking the drugs, also when they get really sick from them? After all, the drugs are supposed to make your feel better, not worse. That comes down for a big part to marketing. The pharmaceutical industry has for a long time been extremely smart with their marketing. They have made us all believe that their products are superior to anything else. They have also infiltrated the universities, so all doctors learn is to treat diseases with pharmaceutical drugs. Doctors know close to nothing about food, herbs, meditation, chiropractic or any other natural treatment. It's not uncommon that doctors just warn their patients that "herbs might harm", "homeopathy is a waste of money" and "chiropractic has not been scientifically proven". They simply don't know that the drugs they prescribe have not been scientifically proven either.

So for the time being we will be stuck with this medical model, though more and more people stop taking drugs. As a result the drug manufacturers push new drugs more and more and don't shy away from inventing diseases to sell drugs. This mainly applies to psychiatric drugs, but it also happens in other areas.
So is there a place for pharmaceuticals in health care? Yes, absolutely. When you have type 1 diabetes you really want insulin and when you get an accident and you have five broken ribs you are very happy to accept painkillers. Surgeons need anaesthetics and at emergency departments some other drugs are very useful. But useful drugs are a very small part of the market. And they should always be the last thing to try, but for most doctors it's the first (and usually only) thing.

Vaccines: a special category
As a last thing I want to say something about an important pharmaceutical product, that most people don't consider drugs. But they are drugs. I'm talking about vaccines. Most of what I have written here about the fraudulent practices of trials and approval

---

[8] "Side effects: death. Confessions of a pharma insider" by John Virapen, chapter 17.

practices doesn't apply to vaccines. For vaccines are not subjected to double blind, placebo controlled trials. They are tested for the ultimate surrogate endpoint: antibodies. If a vaccine is able to produce enough antibodies it's considered effective, even though the antibody story has been debunked decades ago. The safety is tested in very short trials, often not more than two weeks and sometimes even shorter. If children get injected and reactions don't show up within a few days, the vaccine is considered safe. If bad reactions happen a week later, then it's coincidence. Actually, even during the trials most reactions are considered coincidence, which is how the manufacturers can get away with pretty much anything.

And once the very short trials period is over all the manufacturer needs to do is convince the government that this vaccine is absolutely necessary, highly effective and perfectly safe. This is usually a simple job and takes a short period of time. It's a lot easier than getting a normal drug approved. And once the approval is there marketing is hardly necessary. The government will do that job and doctors are also more than willing to push the new shot. And when things go wrong the financial consequences are minimal. Suing the manufacturer of a vaccine in case of death or injury is very hard and in many countries not even possible. The protection is almost absolute. The reason for this strange situation is not easy to explain.

Number one cause of death

Take everything together and it's not hard to imagine why pharmaceuticals are the number one cause of death. Countries that have an obligation for hospitals to report deaths-by-drug have shockingly high numbers for just this. As most drugs are prescribed on an outpatient basis it's impossible to know the real number of drug deaths, but it must be very high. If you then consider the people who die indirectly (e.g. because the drug ruins organs, lowered cholesterol causes heart attacks or anti-depressants cause suicide) then it becomes very hard to understand why this system is still going. The only explanation is the very strong mythology that has been carefully created over the last 100 years. It's hard to convince people that they have been fooled this badly.

6. Obesity

Many books have been written about obesity and thousands of books have been published about how to lose weight. But none of them seem to help against the problem. Doctors tells their patients to lose weight, but have no clue either why the people get so heavy. It's quite embarrassing that many doctors tell the patients how they should change their diets and exercise habits to lose weight. Those patients have likely already tried a few dozen diets and know ten times more about the topic than the doctor. And they also know that nothing works.

So what is really the problem here? All those books, all the studies and all the websites usually focus on two things: diet and exercise. People get overweight because they eat too much, or the wrong things, and they don't exercise enough. The problem is that this is wrong. Of course diet has something to do with it, but forget about the exercise part of the story. Those of you who have looked into this topic know that you need to run for an hour to burn the calories of one hamburger or a few TimTams. And those who do the exercising know that afterwards you are hungry and will easily eat those burnt calories extra in your next meal. Exercising is great for health and fitness. It makes you feel better and if you do it outside you get fresh air. It has loads of benefits, but it won't make you lose weight. Studies have also shown that a year of exercising every day might make you lose 1kg of fat. If you are lucky. Just as many people won't lose any weight at all. Nevertheless most doctors will tell their obese patients to start exercising, as then they will lose weight.

Diet
So we need to focus on the diet, right? Let's see how many myths are going around about diets and obesity.
For a long time we were told that fat is bad for us, because it makes us fat. After all, when we are overweight we carry too much fat, so it's simple: we should eat less fat. This only makes sense when you don't know anything about biochemistry, about metabolism or the human body. Doctors are supposed to know these things and should know it's absurd to say that too much fat makes fat. Unfortunately they have spread this myth for a long time and many are still telling obese patients to limit fat intake. Yes, fat has more calories per

gram, but that's a completely irrelevant number. It is not about the number of calories, but about what your body does with those calories.

So many people started to realise that the "fat makes fat" theory didn't add up and they started to focus on other dietary issues. Many books were written about the low carb diet, with the Atkins diet as the most famous one. Bread got a bad reputation with some people, as did fruits. Vegetables have always been a problem, as they are mainly made of carbohydrates, but few people will say that you shouldn't eat vegetables.

Many people tried the low carb diets and many of them did lose some weight, though not remotely as much as they had hoped for. But it usually came back pretty quickly. And many didn't lose any weight at all. It is pretty obvious that cutting out grains is not the way to lose weight.

But then all the writers of weight loss books came with the answer to all the questions. It wasn't the fat and it wasn't so much the carbs. It was just the sugar! And finally they got a good idea. All the truckloads of sugar are most definitely not good for us and are probably an important reason for the weight gain problems we see everywhere. Usually sugar is seen as "empty calories", but it's a lot more complicated than that. I don't know much about biochemistry, so long lectures or thick books about the effects of sugar are no good for me. But I do understand that sugar is not good for our bodies. It causes all kinds of problems and weight gain is one of them.

So what happened with the obese people who quit the sugar? Most of them lost some weight. Some lost a lot and some didn't lose any. So this was just another failure in the fight against obesity. How on earth is that possible? The science backs this dietary approach, doesn't it? Yes, it does, but only partially.

All the sugar is bad for our health. It causes inflammation, heart disease, diabetes and all kinds of other problems. And it also contributes to obesity. So by all means throw out the sugar. But if you hope to lose 20kg of fat this way you probably will get disappointed.

<u>Surgery</u>
So all the different diets don't make people slim. But doctors are not

discouraged by this. Not only do they keep telling their obese patients that they should change their diets, they also have come with a treatment themselves: lap band surgery. This is a pretty big operation during which a band is put around the stomach, so that it gets much smaller and you can't eat much anymore. This surgery has only negatives. It is a pretty risky operation, it leaves the patient permanently hungry (for the part of the stomach that can't be used will still tell you that it's empty) and when you don't eat much you will get nutrient deficiencies. And does it help? Of course it doesn't, as this is not much else than a very extreme dietary approach. And just like with every diet many patients will lose a certain amount of weight in the beginning, though many don't lose any weight at all. But few are able to keep the weight off. It's just a way to starve yourself and eventually the body might burn the fat that's available (though non-dietary fat reserves might not be touched). But the body has all kinds of protection mechanisms available to prevent starvation. It will use the available energy more and more economically and with little food these people usually start to gain weight again pretty soon after the surgery.

Bariatric surgery is a completely absurd approach of the obesity problem. It's expensive, dangerous and useless. But I'm afraid it won't be abandoned any time soon, as desperate obese people will keep looking for solutions.

What causes obesity?

So what is then the problem and what is the solution? Now it gets complicated, for there are different things that all influence each other. Our bodies are not just a skin with parts inside. We are not machines. We are extremely complicated organisms and everything influences each other in ways that we will never even start to understand. We can only look at some obvious problems.

Obesity has gone out of hand in the last few decades and yes, the consumption of sugar and other junk food has also gone out of hand during that period. But there are also a few other things have got really bad.

The world is being polluted at extremely high speed with many thousands of man-made chemicals and from most of them we have no idea what they will do to us or to other living organisms. But it is known that many of them influence how our bodies work. They can disrupt our hormones, or the way our cells function. And the more there are and the higher the levels, the worse the effect will be. This will be one of the reasons why some people grow heavier and heavier while being on a perfectly healthy diet. And when weight gain isn't caused by food intake, then a change of diet is unlikely to make the fat disappear. Getting rid of chemicals often helps, but it's impossible to create a completely clean living environment. If you search long enough you will probably still find a few places on earth that are quite clean, but it's unlikely you will find even one place that is completely free of nasty chemicals. So any kind of overweight caused by this kind of pollution will be extremely hard to get rid of.

Then there is something else that has gone way out of hand and that's the use of antibiotics. When penicillin was discovered its use pretty soon became widespread. Doctors gave it for everything and anything, from a cold to a sore finger. They knew it didn't work, but it was the magical drug that everyone expected to get and doctors prescribed it generously. They knew it would cause resistance and they knew it killed gut bacteria, but they didn't care. Till it appeared that penicillin didn't work for all bacteria and that many bacteria had developed resistance. Then new antibiotics were developed and their sales exploded. Not only doctors for humans discovered these drugs. Also veterinarians and farmers quickly figured out that it worked for animals. And then they found something else. When animals were treated with antibiotics they would gain weight. The result was that farmers started to routinely give antibiotics to healthy animals, so that they would gain more weight quicker, which meant that the farmer could make more money. Why would anyone think this would be different for humans? Nobody seems to have done any research why antibiotics cause weight gain, but it doesn't matter why it happens. It's a fact that it happens.
It's not unusual nowadays that babies have already had multiple rounds of antibiotics before their first birthday. We really shouldn't be surprised that a few years later they start to get overweight. And again there is a problem with this kind of overweight. Because it's not caused by food intake it won't disappear with a change of diet. Probiotics might help getting the gut bacteria back on track, but that simply doesn't solve the problem. It looks like it's not just the gut bacteria that are involved. There is more to it, but as long as nobody looks into this we won't know. And that means that it's hard to find

the solution.

The best way to deal with this problem is to prevent it. There are plenty of natural antibiotics available, which usually work a lot better, are a lot cheaper and don't cause any health problems. In 10-20 years antibiotics will probably have become useless and if they won't be prescribed anymore, then we might see a decrease in obesity. But that's still far away.

What's more? Again we will have to look at pharmaceuticals. Many drugs cause weight gain and this unwanted effect usually happens in a high number of patients. Especially psychiatric drugs are infamous for this. A high number of people who take anti-depressants or anti-psychotics (and these drugs are prescribed for anything and everything) will experience weight gain. This can be just a few kilograms, but it's not unusual for people to go from a normal weight to obese in a matter of months. And there is a huge problem with this. Once you stop with the drugs the weight usually doesn't disappear. You might lose some of it and some people might lose most of it, but it's not like a few months after stopping you are back on your old weight. So what are these drugs doing to the human metabolism to cause this disaster? I don't think anyone has looked into that. The drugs are popular, are aggressively marketed and doctors prescribe them to anyone who has some problems in life. And the patients get fatter and fatter.

What is the solution?

I'm sure there are more causes of obesity, but I think I have mentioned the most important ones. And a solution does not exist yet. For if anyone would have the solution to obesity this program would become an instant hit and all other weight loss programs would disappear within a few months. Whatever it would be, every obese person would run to it. But nothing really works. The reason is that most approaches are based on diet and even if all the other causes get attention from a practitioner then nobody knows how to deal with it.

This is not a nice or good message, but it's the disastrous reality. Worldwide obesity has become a bigger problem than starvation and every country that adopts the western lifestyle sees an explosion of obesity. And I don't see this stop any time soon. We can change diets, but that's all. We cannot quickly change the amount of toxic chemicals in the environment. We can abandon antibiotics, but that probably won't solve too much of the problem either. The same goes for all the other pharmaceuticals that make people gain weight. For the problem is that whatever we do to our bodies has an influence on our offspring. Whatever all these substances do to the human body, parents will likely pass this on to their children and grandchildren. They will be born with a predisposition to obesity and might not have any chance in escaping this fate.

But there is one thing you can do: stay away from doctors. Not only do they know nothing about obesity, they are the main cause of it. And all they can offer is dangerous and useless treatments. You might not be able to solve your weight problems, but at least you might be able to stop them from getting worse by not taking anything a doctor would prescribe.

7. Cancer

Cancer has become one of the biggest health care problems and it's also the most profitable one. Make no mistake: cancer is a business. Though of course it's impossible to say how much money goes on exactly an educated guess puts it closely to one trillion dollars a year. So you can see why there is a reason for the high number of myths that surround cancer. If people would see all those myths for what they are the cancer industry would likely fall apart.

With some 30% of the population expected to get cancer at some point in life you can imagine that people see it as a problem and many already fear it long before they get a diagnosis. But when you look behind this fear most people are not so much scared for cancer, but for the cancer treatments that usually will follow after the diagnosis. And that's not so strange, for the conventional treatments are horrible. It's a fact that these treatments kill many and I dare to say that most people with cancer die from the cancer diagnosis and the cancer treatment. Few die from the cancer itself.

The more people get cancer, the higher the number of myths.

Myth #1: Cancer is fate.
This is not only completely untrue, but it's also a very dangerous myth. If cancer is your fate and there is nothing you can do to prevent it, then you become helpless. And it's very well known that helpless patients of any disease have a much worse outcome than those who feel in control.

Cancer is not randomly spread out over the population. Those who live in cities are at higher risk than those who live at the countryside. Those who eat junk food are at higher risk than those who prefer vegetables and nuts. Those who have no purpose in life are at higher risk than those who have meaningful activities. Those who feel in control of their bodies and their lives are at much lower risks than those who just do what they are told.

The survival rate of those who choose natural cancer treatments is not only much higher because nature generally doesn't kill, but heals. It's at least as much that those people are in control and they have largely lost their fear. Mind, body and spirit are not separate entities. They aren't even three sides of the same thing. They are one and the same, all integrated. Those who understand that handle disease much better than those who think that disease is just something of the body.

Myth #2: Oncologists know what they are doing.
This is a huge myth. Most people trust their oncologist, for "he's the doctor and he knows what's best". Reality is that oncologists know very little about cancer. I know that sounds odd, but it's true. You could pretty easily find that out if you would ask an oncologist a series of basic questions.
- Where does cancer come from?
- Why does someone get cancer at a certain place and not somewhere else?
- How often does cancer disappear on its own?
- Could there be a specific reason why the body develops cancer?
- How many false positives do your tests give?
- If cancer spreads, why does it usually spread to the other side of the body and not to a nearby place?
- Could cancer be a systemic disease? If so, why don't you treat it as such?
- What is the cure rate of your treatments?
- What is the cure rate of proper natural treatments?
- How many patients live longer as a result of your treatments and how many live shorter?
- How do you determine life expectancy?
Any of these questions will get you no answer or a very vague answer. They don't know what they are talking about. They just follow the protocols that they have been taught at university. They can see that the treatments don't work, but that doesn't stop them. In some countries chemotherapy is very profitable for the oncologists, but in many countries they have nothing to gain from it. And still they have their treatment rooms filled with people who get chemo. If they would know what they are doing they would never ever give anyone this stuff.

It's quite simple. If you want to know about cancer an oncologist is the last person to go to.

Myth #3: a lot more people survive cancer nowadays.

Oncology loves smokescreens and they are masters in manipulating data. First of all there is the word "survive". Oncologists generally don't talk about cure, they talk about "five years survival". Most people think that that means "five years cancer free", but that's not true. It simply means that five years after the initial diagnosis you are still alive. You could be full of tumours and you might die three weeks later, but you are still a "survivor". Here is also the explanation for why screening programs work so well. If you can find cancer two years earlier it will be much easier to reach that five years line. But it doesn't have any influence whatsoever on your life expectancy.

Something oncology also likes to hide is that most cancers don't grow that quickly and even if you don't do anything whatsoever many people would easily live another five years. It has even been proven that the average cancer patient who does nothing lives 3-4 times as long as the ones that accept conventional treatment. Still oncologists love to scare their patients saying that "if you don't get treatment you will die soon". Oncologists are very bad in determining life expectancy anyway, which is not so strange, considering they have no idea what they are talking about.

The term "survival" is necessary to hide the abysmal results of conventional cancer treatments. People might think that it means cure, but it couldn't be further away from the truth.

> Cure: if after the last treatment your chances of getting a certain medical condition is the same as for the general population.

Oncologists don't cure anyone and they know it. They know that most patients get another cancer diagnosis. They know that their treatments are one of the main causes of cancer. That's why they use the smokescreen term "survival".

But what about all those people who survive cancer nowadays? Cancer organisations love to point out how many people survive certain types of cancer. But again we are dealing with a smokescreen. Every time you get a new cancer diagnosis you will go into the statistics as a new cancer patient. It's not unusual for someone to get three or more separate cancer diagnoses. But you can only die once. So you might survive breast cancer and lung cancer, just to die from pancreatic cancer three years later. But this way the statistics for breast and lung cancer look much better.
Reality is that more people than ever get cancer and more people than ever die from it (directly or indirectly).

Myth 4: Conventional treatments are the best way to treat cancer.

I find it hard to understand that this myth is still going so strong. With so many cancer patients everyone knows someone who had cancer and they know how horrible the treatments are. And they know that it didn't help and their friend, neighbour or relative died anyway. The only explanation I can think of is that people are scared of dying and oncologists are very skilled in scaring their patients into accepting treatments. "If you don't get the treatments, then you will die soon" is a very common way of talking. It's usually not true.

Surgery, radiation and chemotherapy don't cure. There are people who stay alive for a long time, but that is in spite of and not thanks to the treatments. Reality is that about 2% of those who accept conventional cancer treatments get cured. But don't be fooled by this percentage. As oncologists have no idea what they are talking about there is a significant number of false positives. How high this number is remains unclear, but I have heard oncologists admit in front of the camera that for breast cancer the percentage is at least 10%. For other types of cancer this might be higher or lower. But these people only need to survive the treatments to be "cured" of a cancer they didn't have in the first place. It's also known that many cancers disappear on their own, so if these people hadn't had treatment they would also have been cured. And of course there are the growing number of people who have been given up by their oncologists and then start looking for alternatives. If they cure themselves with natural treatments they will still go into the statistics as cured from cancer. If you take these numbers you can only come to the conclusion that not only do conventional treatments not cure anyone, they actually kill loads of people who could have lived a long life if they had stayed away from oncologists.

And these numbers are not wild guesses. They are based on scientific research, admissions of oncologists and a bit of common sense.

Myth #5: Natural treatments have not been proven to work.
Let's first state that it has been proven that conventional treatments don't work. They don't work in a lab and they don't work in real life. They don't work in theory and they don't work in reality. They just don't work. That means that when someone chooses to treat cancer with natural therapies they have nothing to lose. But conventional treatments kill a high number of patients and natural treatments are safe. So it should be a no-brainer what to choose. But unfortunately loads of people refuse to even look into natural treatments, because "there is no proof that they work".

So what is the definition of proof? It should work in a lab and it should work in real life. If that is the definition of proof many natural (or alternative) cancer treatment have an abundance of proof of efficacy. But you won't read about this in mainstream media, for the cancer industry does not like this of course. Remember: they have a trillion dollars a year to lose. For such amounts you will do more than keep silent about facts.

So what happens if someone is diagnosed with cancer, but refuses conventional treatments? Even if they keep going to the doctor for regular tests, then still the person likely won't go into the statistics. So if you cure your cancer you will simply not show up anywhere. It's like you never had cancer. That's why there is no statistical proof that natural treatments work. And if you had all conventional treatments before you go natural, then these treatments will officially be the ones that cured you, even if the oncologist said that it hadn't worked. Just as the statistics are manipulated to make conventional treatments look good, so are they manipulated to make natural treatments look bad.

Many books have been written about how to treat cancer naturally, so I don't see a need to repeat that information here.[9] There are literally hundreds of ways to cure cancer and many treatments are very cheap. Many people can cure their cancer for just a few hundred dollars.

Myth #6: a good test result means you are cancer free.
Oncologists know this is a myth. They know that scans and blood tests are meaningless, which is the reason why they tell the patients to keep coming back every couple of months for new scans and new tests. That's why they generally don't tell their patients "you are cured", but "the test results don't show up any cancer cells". They know that this only means that the tests don't show up any cancer cells and nothing more than that. The tests are useless and say absolutely nothing about the future. Still patients of course believe that this is really good. Even if after a certain period of time the tests are still good, then you won't be told that you are cured. You are "in remission", which is another smokescreen term. Oncologists know that almost all patients come back sooner or later to get another cancer diagnosis. The remission can last a month, a year, or a few years, but rarely longer than that.

Myth #7: tumours can metastasise and spread to other places in the body.
This theory sounds good. You have breast cancer and a year later you have bone cancer, so hasn't it just spread? But why then do oncologists treat one cancer differently than another? They say that it makes a huge difference where the tumour is. That contradicts each other. And if tumour cells would start wandering, then you would expect that the second cancer would be leukaemia or lymphoma. At least you would expect it at a place close to the first tumour. But it's usually somewhere totally different.

Reality is that the first and the second cancer have nothing to do with each other. The second one is simply a new tumour. That's not strange, as cancer is a systemic disease and not a local one. There are all kinds of reasons why you get a specific type of cancer, but one doesn't exclude the other. On top of that the conventional cancer treatments are known to be highly carcinogenic. Actually, cancer

---

[9] Books I recommend are "Cancer free" by Bill Henderson and "Outsmart your cancer" by Tanya Harter Pierce. Also the website https://thetruthaboutcancer.com/ is very useful.

treatments are the nr. 1 cause of cancer. This is how oncologists keep themselves in a job. There is no business like return business.

And here you have the reason why people who treat cancer naturally usually don't get a second diagnosis. They have changed their attitude and usually their lifestyle and diet. And they have avoided the main cause of cancer.

Myth #8: Early detection saves lives.

Fact: early detection only makes good statistics. As I already said: if you detect a tumour early your chances of living another five years are simply bigger. It's nothing but simple mathematics. It doesn't make you live one day longer.

On the contrary. When you participate in screening programs and a tumour is detected you most probably will get talked into immediate treatment with surgery, radiation and/or chemotherapy. These treatments have a high mortality rate, which means that you die a lot earlier than if you hadn't been diagnosed. Screening programs also cause a high number of false positives, so quite a few people are killed by cancer treatments when they never had cancer at all. That's not what you are told when screening programs are advertised. And last but not least: the screenings are not harmless. Mammograms are known to cause cancer. Bowel cancer screening often sends people for a colonoscopy, which is a risky procedure. Skin cancer screening might not kill you, but often pieces are cut out and that leaves you mutilated. Prostate cancer tests often lead to biopsies, which have a high risk of infection.

If you have health problems, or you feel a tumour, then it's a good idea to get a diagnosis. As long as you stay away from conventional cancer treatments, as they will kill you. If you use natural treatments early detection won't really give you a better chance for a cure, for these treatments can cure in at least 99% of the cases anyway. But at an earlier stage it's faster and easier and you have more time to find the treatment that works for you.

So why do oncologists what they do?

That's a very good question, but one that doesn't have a general answer. Oncologists are at a long distance the type of doctors that kill the most of their patients. And they know it. It's not possible that they don't know it, as they see it daily in their practice. So are all oncologists evil murderers? Of course not. That would be way too easy. I know that in the USA (and possibly other countries) oncologists can make a lot of money by selling chemotherapy to their patients. That makes their recommendations and motives highly questionable. But in many countries oncologists don't make any more money whether they prescribe radiation and chemo or not. Surgeries are profitable for almost all surgeons, but oncologists don't always do the surgeries themselves. But even if the doctors have no financial interest in the treatments they usually still do the same things.

Assuming these people do not enjoy torturing and killing their patients, it's a mystery why they do this. I suppose they tell themselves that this is the best that can be done. It's how they have been trained and once you are in the system it's not easy to get out. If you want to know the reasons for oncologists to butcher, burn and poison their patients, then you will have to ask them. But I doubt you will get an answer.

8. Tests

A hundred years ago doctors didn't have much else to diagnose disease than their knowledge, common sense and questions. Doctors asked the patient loads of questions and after 15 minutes they had a pretty good idea what was wrong with the person. Not anymore. Doctors still ask questions, but they are mainly focused on figuring out what kind of test would be the most appropriate. And it's not so rare that a doctor asks hardly any questions at all and prints a test form within two minutes. Most doctors don't dare or are not able to diagnose any disease anymore without using tests. So as these tests are so important in the medical practice you would assume that they are really good and accurate and therefore very important. But that's far away from the truth.

Lab tests

Tests go from simple lab tests, to x-rays and all kinds of scans and procedures to look into the body. I don't know how accurate doctors think these tests are, but from some they are well aware that the accuracy is poor. Let's start with the basic lab test. If you look at the results you will see a range of values and whatever is within that range is assumed to be normal. That range is often huge, so what on earth is normal? If the range of test X is 3-8 and your value is 7.9, then that's normal. If the value is 8.1, then at once you have a problem. Those numbers are way too static and as doctors only look at the test results and are not trained to think about such details the result of a any lab test becomes unreliable and nothing more than an indication that something might be right or wrong. Nevertheless the waiting rooms of blood collection centres are usually full and whole treatment plans are based on the results of lab tests.

Scans

So what about scans? There are all kinds of them. CAT scans, MRI scans, PET scans, SPECT scans, ultrasounds and I probably miss a few. Considering the importance of these tests you would assume they are highly accurate. And they are, in a certain way. They are accurate in the picture they provide to the doctor, but that picture needs to be interpreted and that is where things get shaky. Doctors are like programmed robots and are generally not able to think outside the box. They have learnt that a certain picture has a certain meaning and that's about it. But what if the meaning of a picture is actually different? Then they are usually unable to see the discrepancy. If a patient has every symptom of MS, but the MRI scan doesn't show what it should show, then the doctor won't diagnose MS. On the other hand, most people show abnormalities on a spinal X-ray, even when they don't have any back problems whatsoever. Obviously those abnormalities are not abnormal at all, but still doctors make diagnoses based on those X-rays. Many doctors are aware that spinal X-rays are useless, but they get then done anyway, because printing test forms is the only thing they know. It's the idea that a useless test is better than no test and with that they have elevated tests to the level of main diagnostic tool, though tests should at best be support to help diagnosing.

A look inside
So what about these procedures to look into the body? Doctors nowadays have all kinds of viewing tools and those tests sound really impressive. But the results only mean something if the doctor knows what he's looking at and there it often goes wrong. Many "abnormal" knees are perfectly fine and many "sick" bowels are actually healthy. When doctors can't differentiate between normal and abnormal and don't understand that every person is unique, then such procedures become largely meaningless. People even get operated just to see if there is something wrong. But whatever the doctor finds, he often doesn't know whether this is the cause of the problem or not.

The costs of testing
If all that testing would be harmless, it would only cost a lot of money, but that would be it. But of course that's not remotely true. First of all, many tests come with a risk. The lab test is generally safe, but most scans use radio-active radiation, which for a long time has been known to be dangerous. 40 years ago the general advice was to limit X-rays as much as possible for that reason. But then the CT-scan was introduced and quickly became widely used. CT scanners use a much higher level of radiation and soon it was forgotten that X-rays are dangerous. So doctors nowadays prescribe X-rays like they are as safe as a urine test. And CT scans are routinely ordered, even if there is little justification for it. MRI scanners use magnetism, which is also harmful (why do you think

you are alone in the room?) Ultrasounds seem to be pretty safe for adults, but not for babies. It is amazing how quickly the pregnancy ultrasound became the standard, when there was absolutely no proof that this was safe. X-rays for pregnant women were once assumed to be safe and it took doctors a very long time to accept that they were not safe at all. Proof is emerging that ultrasounds are not safe for the unborn baby either, though at this moment it's not clear how dangerous these scans are exactly.

That's only the risks of the tests themselves, but at least as dangerous is the treatment the patient often gets as the result of a test. "This is the test result and so this is the treatment" is usually the standard approach from doctors. The treatment is usually drugs or surgery, for doctors don't know much else. So loads of people get drugs for non-existing diseases or undergo completely unnecessary surgeries. When you realise that 20% of the appendices taken out are perfectly healthy (do you also wonder why they cut them out?) and 85% of the people have abnormal spinal X-rays (which not rarely leads to surgery) you see the problem. And many people get immediately a prescription for blood pressure lowering medication when the instruments show elevated pressure during the first visit. It's perfectly normal for blood pressure to be high in the doctor's room, as most people are at least slightly stressed.

Doctors don't want to know how useless most of their tests are, as they are helpless without them. They can't diagnose measles or flu anymore without a lab test, though also those tests are highly unreliable. Measuring blood pressure is almost a standard ritual, no matter what you come in for. Take away all the equipment and the printer for test forms and most doctors are totally helpless. Well, they can still Google your symptoms, but you can also do that yourself. But when you self-diagnose you aren't taken seriously by anyone. For not only doctors are completely dependent on tests, most patients also feel that a diagnosis is only real when they have had tests.

So if you consider getting tests done, ask yourself if there is any use to it. The use of most tests is limited and the risks are real. In many cases you are better off without. And it also saves a lot of money.

9. The brain

Our skull gives space to one of the biggest mysteries on earth: the brain. We know that the brain is made up of grey matter and we know a few things about the structure. The technical details are pretty easy to find with autopsies on dead bodies. But that doesn't mean that doctors have any idea what those things mean. They pretend that they know a lot about the brain, but it's generally not much more than assumptions. Neurologists (the doctors that deal with the brain and nerve system) love brain scans, because they can make impressive statements about what disease someone has or doesn't have. But in most cases this is not based on anything.

MRI scans

Neurologists have a variety of diagnostic tools, which they use a lot. Often these tests have little to offer and just cause a lot of confusion, but the machines are there and will be used. It gives validity to a diagnosis and the patients want that scientific confirmation nowadays.

MRI scanners are very popular. Google "MRI scan" and you will see a variety of colourful pictures, which all are supposed to tell us something about the brain of the person in the scanner. But if you start to dig deeper then those pictures don't have that much value. They can register if there is electrical activity in a certain part of the brain, but that's all. What does it mean if there is high or low electrical activity somewhere in your grey matter? Is it good or bad? That is open to interpretation and it usually depends on the disease symptoms the patient displays. The problem is that MRI scans are expensive and the scanners are pretty scarce. So usually only people with neurological symptoms will get a scan. But to get a better idea of what those pictures mean you would have to scan large numbers of perfectly healthy people. That's not only practically impossible, but all scans can be dangerous and you cannot expose many healthy people to these risks just for research. So how many healthy people walk around on earth with brains that show the electrical activity of someone with a severe neurological disease? Nobody knows.

The problem with doctors is that they can't think beyond what they have learned and they adjust their diagnosis based on a test. This is an explanation for the exploding number of diagnoses for diseases that seem to be very similar. If doctors would have an open mind there wouldn't be a lot left of their theories about the brain. Let's assume that patient X has all the symptoms of multiple sclerosis. The neurologist will put him into an MRI scanner and the pictures don't show what the doctor expects to see. The conclusion of the doctor will be that the person doesn't have MS and he will come up with an alternative diagnosis. But a more logical conclusion would be that the interpretation of the MRI scan is wrong. And this way many very sick people are told that there is nothing wrong with them and that they should see a psychiatrist. Or they get a diagnosis that fits the scan, but not the symptoms. Or they are told that they have a "MS like disease" (whatever name they give it). Anything will be done not to admit that their fancy scanners are useless.

CT scans
But what about CT scans? They show clearly what's wrong, don't they? Well, they show structural pictures of the brain, but they don't tell what they mean. If you have a lesion in a part of the brain, does that mean you are sick? Does that mean there is something wrong? Maybe you have had that lesion for 20 years, but you didn't know because you didn't get the CT scan. And here you see the same problem that MRI scans have: you don't know what the scans would say about the person's brain before they got sick. Maybe this specific picture is perfectly normal for this person and not the cause of disease. It's known that some 85% of the people have abnormalities in their spines without them causing backaches. Couldn't that be the same with the brain? That is actually quite likely.

Another problem for the whole brain theory is the handful of people in the world who have hardly any brain activity whatsoever, but still function normally. Nobody can explain that, as we know that brain injury (e.g. after an accident) can cause loads of problems. The only correct conclusion from this is that we have no clue how the brain really works. But that would be way too inconvenient, so this kind of information is usually ignored. Neurologists stick with what they can see and what they can interpret and simply ignore everything that doesn't fit their theories. It's obvious that this is a recipe for disaster. Doctors are hardly the most competent profession, but neurologists just make guesses and then they dress up their guesses as "evidence based medicine".

Curing brain damage

But those people who have got the brain injuries really do have permanent damage, right? Neurologists usually tell such patients that there isn't much they can do about it and they need to live with it. They also tell that to patients with neurological diseases. But it's not true. These doctors just don't keep up with their reading or are too lazy to do so. Or too arrogant. The body has a very big ability to self-healing and the brain isn't that much different.

More and more stories are surfacing of people with a variety of neurological diseases and damage who managed to largely cure themselves, simply by retraining the brain. There is no surgery and no drugs involved, though researchers do now and then invent machines that help patients with this retraining. When one area of the brain is damaged it is often possible for other areas of the brain to take over that function. Most neurologists don't know this and stick with the old story that brains are parted into neat areas and once there is damage that's it. But that's obviously not true. And these new discoveries aren't even in the area of alternative treatments, but they are done in the accepted scientific way. So it's strange that so many neurologists stick with what clearly has shown to be incorrect. So how does this retraining work? I would say that that doesn't really matter, but for many people that's not a satisfactory answer. They absolutely want to know how it's possible that brain damage can be cured by the patient. But the answer is that nobody knows.

Reality is that the brain is a thousand times more complicated than we will ever understand and that's where we should start with any kind of research. The whole idea that we do know what the brain is and how it functions is very dangerous, because it leads to simplification of something extremely complicated. And as a result many mistakes are made, obvious problems are ignored and patients are sent home without hope. And doctors keep filling people up with drugs and vaccines that cannot possibly have been tested for potential brain damage. It's simple: keep all toxic substances out of your body, so that they can't reach the brain. For you really want to keep your grey cells healthy.

10. Dementia

In the late 1800's age related dementia was very rare, which was the reason that Alois Alzheimer first properly described the disease in 1901. Many people will say that this was because people didn't get that old, but that's a very stubborn myth. Indeed in the 1800's the average age in western countries was pretty low. This was caused by high infant mortality and poor living circumstances for the lowest class (which was a big proportion of the population). When you live on the garbage heap and drink from the sewer it's not too likely that you will make it to 60. But those who lived in reasonably good conditions, who had enough food and clean water easily made it to 80, 90 or even 100 years old. Still they didn't develop dementia. So let's forget about the theory that dementia is a normal part of old age. It's not.

So what is the medical description of dementia? Now it gets interesting. When doctors talk about all their different diagnoses they sound like they know what they are talking about, but in reality they are just making guesses. The cause of dementia is assumed to be in the brain, so when a patient shows symptoms doctors will do brain scans. When someone has "plaques" and "holes in the brain" the patient will be diagnosed with Alzheimer's disease. But there are a lot of problems with this theory.

Diagnosing
Alzheimer's disease is labelled as a specific type of dementia and it should come with certain behaviour. So what happens if someone has the "correct" brain scans, but not the behaviour that is "typical" for Alzheimer's disease? I have experienced that personally, when long ago my mother developed dementia. She had the plaques and the holes, but not the typical Alzheimer symptoms. So she was diagnosed with atypical Alzheimer's disease. I never understood what that was and I still don't know. It's a "we have no idea" kind of diagnosis and it shows the lack of facts behind it. So were the scans she got of any use? Obviously not, for it didn't make any difference. Medical treatment wasn't available anyway.

But then there is the situation that someone meets all the criteria for

Alzheimer's disease, but the brain scans do not show plaques. Nowadays doctors can't think for themselves anymore, but completely rely on their tests. When the observations, theories and test results don't line up they simply invent a new diagnosis. And so many dementia patients are labelled with vascular dementia. I had to look up how this type of dementia is diagnosed and all I found was a heap of tests that can be done, but no clear criteria. It seems that this type of dementia is again a label that says "we don't really know, but you don't meet the criteria for Alzheimer's." Interesting is that it's generally recognised that there is a lot of overlap between the different types of dementia, making the labels (and the tests) even less useful.

Then there is Lewy body dementia, which is assumed to be caused by problems in the neurons and it's considered a neurological disease. And if none of these diagnoses really fits, then there is always the option to blame other diseases, or viruses, or genes for it.

Religious Orders Study
In the 1990's the Religious Orders Study was done. A high number of older nuns, monks and priests had agreed to get tests for cognitive functioning and after they died from old age their brains could be examined. The results were interesting. It appeared that many of these people had brains full of plaques and other problems, but in life they hadn't had any cognitive problems. This means that the plaques are not characteristic for dementia and might not have anything to do with it whatsoever. Maybe many young people also have these plaques in their brains. Maybe they go again after a while? Maybe they are related to lifestyle and disappear again if you change your diet, or stress levels, or other factors. Of course the doctors won't even think about this, as they have decided that plaques are the thing to diagnose Alzheimer's disease.

It would be interesting to know how many young people have such brains, but we won't know. Many younger people who die from any cause end up at the autopsy table, but the pathologists won't look at plaques in the brain and if they would see it they wouldn't write it down. Though such things would provide very valuable information it can also be a career killer and doctors don't like to take that risk. Too many doctors who dared to point out flaws in theories disappeared into anonymity. So whatever is really happening in the brains of people of all ages we will probably never know. And doctors keep doing their fancy brain scans to diagnose dementia, even though this has obviously no value.

Real causes

Here you also get the huge problems with scientific research after the cause of dementia and possibly treatments. Whenever you read about such studies you will notice that everything focuses on these theories, which have never been proven to be correct and are very likely incorrect. Researchers look for proteins that cause the plaques and for genes that cause blood vessels to pop. It's not so strange that that kind of research never produces any results. For this long Religious Orders Study so far hasn't produced any useful outcomes. The theory is that people with a "dementia brain", but no cognitive problems, have some kind of back up that they can use. But what the researchers should really focus on is why dementia is so common, when it was so rare 100 years ago. (Obviously it's not genetic.) And why it's so common in the western world and quite rare in other areas. Obviously there are environmental factors that cause the problem. If researchers would forget about their scans and look at other factors, then answers would probably not be so hard to find. Almost every disease is systematic; it involves the whole body and not just one organ. There is no reason to think that dementia is any different.

It's quite likely that inflammation plays a role, as it plays a role in many diseases that are so common nowadays and are closely linked to the western lifestyle. Chronic inflammation is a new phenomenon and it's largely caused by bad diets and a variety of toxic substances that shouldn't be in our bodies.
Countries that culturally consume a lot of turmeric (a powerful anti-inflammatory) have very low incidence of dementia (from all diagnoses). That's not scientific evidence, but it simply makes a lot of sense.

11. Psychiatry

Psychiatry has a chequered past. Insane people have probably always existed and for a long time they were simply locked up in asylums and were forgotten. The asylums were the places where psychiatrists started their profession, but they weren't the only ones who worked there. They had a lot of competition from other specialists, especially neurologists. I'm not sure how these people got their titles, as official medical schools were still in their infancy. I assume that everyone just did what they liked and gave themselves a title based on their interests. Sigmund Freud was not a psychiatrist, but a neurologist, who developed the theories of psycho-analysis.

The doctors in the asylums couldn't do much for their patients. They never cured one and their treatments had little effect. For that reason other doctors considered psychiatrists not-quite-doctors, which the psychiatrists didn't like. So they invented all kinds of treatments, which they said would cure their patients. But that never happened. Most of those treatments were highly torturous and many patients died from them. The theory that insanity was located in the brain already dates from the 1800's and it led to all kinds of horrible treatments. Most of those are largely forgotten, but many still remember the lobotomy, where an ice pick was stuck through the eye to destroy a part of the brain. It was just as barbaric as all the previous surgical interventions and just as useless. It's hard to imagine that the inventor got a Nobel Prize for this, but a lot of Nobel prizes for medicine have been awarded for procedures that have long been abandoned. This is a strong indication for the lack of real science in medicine.
Electroshocks were another barbaric treatment, meant to "fry" parts of the brain, which was supposed to cure mental health problems. It was also completely useless and it's therefore really frightening that this treatment is still used. It's now called "electro convulsive therapy", but it's just the same as 100 years ago. The only difference is that nowadays drugs are used to make the patient limp, so that the arms and legs don't shock so unsightly. It's just as bad for the patient, but much easier for the doctors and nurses.

When pharmaceuticals became mainstream in doctor's offices psychiatrists again missed out, because they didn't have anything to prescribe. But that changed in the early 1900's. Heroin and cocaine appeared to be very useful, but highly addictive, so doctors stopped prescribing those drugs. But after that one drug after another came and all either killed the patients or made them addicted and none of them actually cured anyone. All those older drugs have disappeared from the market again, but till that happened the manufacturers made neat amounts of money with them.

The manual

During the mid 1900's psychiatry slowly started to move from asylums to ordinary doctor's offices and with that psychiatrists got finally the status of real doctors, with a prescription pad on their desks. And then they got help from the American Psychiatric Association, which in 1953 published its first Diagnostic and Statistic Manual of Mental Disorders (DSM). There are no statistics in this book. That word has just been added to give it credibility. The book is filled with a variety of psychiatric diagnoses and descriptions of symptoms. All psychiatrists need to do is look in the book and find a diagnosis that fits the story of the patient. The book has now its 5th edition and with every new edition a number of diagnoses was added. As the number of psychiatrists increased quickly this was a very helpful tool. But to keep all those doctors busy new diagnoses had to be added, so that more people could qualify for a psychiatric label. For with the DSM also the number of psychiatric drugs started to increase rapidly.

You would think that a manual that is so popular is based on scientific evidence, but nothing could be further from the truth. In this book I explain why most of the conventional medical system is not particularly "evidence based", but psychiatry is really outdoing all other areas of medicine. For nothing in the DSM is based on science or evidence. Everything is observations, ideas, opinions and a lot of fancy fantasies. Psychiatrists don't have a lab test or a scan to diagnose any disease. All they have is the DSM with diagnostic criteria. The result is that a patient with exactly the same story might get five different diagnoses from five different psychiatrists.

Of course there is a gigantic problem with this approach. Psychiatrists can do whatever they want and nobody can prove that they are wrong, as nobody can prove that they are correct. And they can invent new diagnoses whenever they want. For the DSM has grown enormously. The exact number of diagnoses is a bit unclear, as it depends on how you count. There are loads of sub-diagnoses and sub-sub-diagnoses, but the number is somewhere between 150-300. The latest version has a lot of diagnoses that end with NOS: Not Otherwise Specified. That means something like "we have decided that there is something wrong with you, but we don't know yet how to define it". Whenever you see the letters NOS you know you are dealing with a weird psychiatric label.

So where do these new diagnoses come from? As there is no diagnostic test, how do psychiatrists decide that there is a new disease or disorder? Well, they vote on it. A group of psychiatrists come together and some propose a new diagnosis. This is discussed and then voted on and that's it. Most votes count and a new disease is added to the list. If you think that this is absurd you are correct. Still somehow the profession manages to make it sound like this is all very scientific and that has a lot of problems.

Opinions
Psychiatrists are often used in courts to determine whether someone should be sent to prison or not. When you are declared insane you are usually sent to a psychiatric facility for treatment. But how does anyone decide whether you are cured and can be released into society? There are no tests, so you completely rely on the opinion of psychiatrists.

It's also becoming more and more common for children and teenagers to get diagnosed with mental health issues. Children are often excluded from school because they have ADHD and won't be allowed back unless they take medication. So children miss out on education based on a diagnosis that was invented and voted on.

So what are psychiatrists doing? While talk therapy once was a more or less important part of psychiatric practice, most psychiatrists don't do much of this anymore. They leave that to psychologists, which of course are lower in rank, as they are not doctors. Though often confused, psychologists are therapists and psychiatrists are doctors, with the full basic medical training. Psychologist cannot prescribe drugs, though some are happy to tell you to ask your doctor for this or that drug.

Though some psychiatrists still include some talk therapy in their treatments, most nowadays mainly prescribe drugs. How long it takes to get a prescription depends on the country and the individual psychiatrist. Many don't mind handing out prescriptions after just one 15 minutes consultation. I suppose these people have learnt the DSM by heart and can easily throw around labels. And for every label there is a drug.

Drugs

There are loads of psychiatric drugs available, as they are an easy way to make money for the pharmaceutical industry. For whatever drug they have they can match a number in the DSM and then start marketing it to the doctors. And doctors prescribe. Not only psychiatrists, but unfortunately many GP's are also very easy in prescribing these very heavy drugs like they are aspirins. Pharmaceutical representatives also heavily target GP's, as their number of patients is much higher than what psychiatrists have. So GP's now start to diagnose people with ADHD, depression, anxiety, bi-polar disorder or whatever is a popular diagnosis. And the patients walk out with a prescription for a drug, instead of a referral to a psychologist or the advice to take a holiday.

Psychiatric drugs usually target the brain in one way or another. Considering how little is known about the brain this is a very dangerous practice. And it's not like the drugs cure anyone. At best they suppress symptoms (but that goes for almost all drugs), while turning the patients into zombies or addicts. For while opioid painkillers get a lot of bad publicity because they can sometimes be addictive, it's psychiatric drugs that are the real problem. Anti-depressants are prescribed like they are as harmless as a cup of tea, but many people find out that these drugs are not only very unpleasant, but that it's often very hard to quit them. There are stories of people who just can't stop, because no matter what they do, lowering the dose sends them into psychosis. That doesn't sound like drugs that should be prescribed in a GP's office to someone who has trouble handling the problems of daily life, but it happens on a daily basis. Many doctors have become a bit more careful with prescribing benzodiazepines (tranquillisers like Valium), but they seamlessly moved on prescribing anti-depressants, which are at least as bad. But also very heavy anti-psychotic drugs are prescribed like they are harmless, often off label to patients without psychosis, who then immediately get a mental health mark in their medical file. And once you have that mark it can be very hard to get rid of it.

Cures
So does psychiatry have any value? Maybe, but it's not much. Psychiatric diseases do exist. Schizophrenia is not a new diagnosis and depression also existed in the past, but then it was called melancholia. And there are some other things that are real. But does that mean that psychiatrists can do anything? No, they can't. The whole history of psychiatry is one of failures. If you have problems with life (which psychiatrists and other doctors love to label as "mental health issues"), then go to a psychologist, a minister, a friend or neighbour, or just wait till things improve. If you have real psychiatric issues, then natural approaches are often remarkably effective. For in contrast with the medical doctrines, psychiatric problems are not located in the brain, but in the gut. A change of diet, vitamins or other supplements and other natural approaches have cured many patients. A naturopath is a lot better than a psychiatrist and they won't give you anything that kills you.

12. HIV/AIDS

The story of AIDS starts in the USA in the early 1980's. A bit of background for this is important. The American CDC (Centers for Disease Control) and NIH (National Institute of Health) had a hard time staying alive. There were two reasons for this. Polio had been "eradicated", measles didn't scare anyone anymore, vaccines weren't pushed aggressively yet and basically there wasn't much work left for these agencies. Another reason was the swine flu hype of 1976. For no reason at all the CDC and NIH announced that a disastrous swine flu epidemic was going to happen. A vaccine was quickly developed and pushed on the public, but this vaccine appeared to be very dangerous and it killed and injured many. The compensation claims got very expensive. And worst of all: the swine flu never happened, let alone that it was an epidemic. This very badly affected the reputation of the CDC and NIH and they were in desperate need of something to give them credibility again.

And then there was AIDS and soon after that there was HIV. That was a very nice coincidence for both government agencies. I don't like coincidences any more than I like conspiracy theories, so you can decide yourself what you think about this.

The first patients
The first AIDS patients were American gay men in their 30's and 40's. They developed what became the "hallmark" of AIDS: Kaposi sarcoma (KS), a skin condition, and pneumocystis pneumonia (PCP), a fungal disease of the lungs. At that time virology was already an area of science that came with a lot of funding, work, fame and prestige, so it was quickly decided that these guys had an infectious disease. That none of the initial patients knew each other was overlooked.

And something else was completely ignored. These guys had been active in the "gay party scene" for a long time. Among those men the use of drugs was standard and especially "poppers" (alkyl nitrites) were very popular, because these drugs make anal sex more pleasant. But it's dangerous stuff and it destroys the blood vessels in the long term. The use of poppers became popular in the early 1970's and it takes about ten years of regular use before the damage shows up. KS is entirely caused by damage caused by poppers. When the blood vessels break down from the inside fungi come in to clear up the debris and so it's not so strange that PCP showed up as well. Retrospectively the "AIDS" symptoms were completely predictable and nobody should have been surprised. Doctors should have told these guys "I warned you that would happen", but they didn't make the connection.

What about the poor immune systems these guys had? Because of the sex with unlimited partners these men had so many venereal diseases that many doctors put them on permanent antibiotics. Antibiotics are toxic and destroy your gut flora, which severely impairs your immune system. Antibiotic overuse can also stimulate fungal overgrowth. And as I said, poppers were not the only drugs these people used. Many of them used pretty much any recreational drug on the market.

So now you might wonder how it's possible that this all was completely overlooked. The connection was too obvious to miss.

HIV
Nevertheless the search for a virus started and the disease was changed from GRID (Gay Related Immune Deficiency) to AIDS (Acquired Immune Deficiency Syndrome). The name AIDS was not incorrect. The disease was acquired (you are not born with it), it came with immune deficiency and the syndrome part was added to have a lot of space to add whatever the officials wanted. But this name went completely out of hand once a virus was "discovered". The discovery of HIV was surrounded by fraud, deception, wishful thinking, fantasy and ambitions. Science was largely absent. The story is very complex and this book is not the place to repeat all this.[10] Simply said: there is no HIV virus. As I explained earlier in this book, virology is a hoax in its entirety. HIV is not an exception. The existence of an AIDS causing virus has never remotely been established.

The viral story has a lot of problems anyway. If a healthy immune system can handle any virus, then why can't it attack HIV? And why

[10] If you want to know all the details I refer you to the books "Fear of the Invisible" by Janine Roberts and "Virus mania" by Torsten Engelbrecht and Claus Köhnlein.

does the virus stay dormant for years before it causes disease? This goes for any "dormant virus". How does a virus cause your immune system to break down? Either the immune system is already very bad or it eliminates the virus. And HIV infection is proven with an antibody test. But antibodies were always said to be protective against disease. If you have a high antibody count against e.g. measles you are told that you are immune to measles. But if you have a high HIV antibody count you are told that you will die. You can't have your cake and eat it.

The test
Of course the whole story of AIDS hangs on the result of a test. (Well, not really, as I will explain later). If you don't have a positive HIV test you can't get AIDS. But this test is a weird one. A very weird one. First of all this test comes with a questionnaire about your lifestyle and medical history, for the results of a HIV test need to be interpreted. Can you imagine getting a cancer biopsy or a blood sugar test and the results depend on your risk factors? It's absurd, but nobody complains.

But it gets worse. When a lab test is done you expect that a test kit is used that is suitable for the test you are getting done. Not so for HIV. When you Google it you can find examples of test kit inserts. Two examples.

Abbott Real Time HIV-1 test insert states: "This assay is not intended to be used as a screening test for HIV-1 or as a diagnostic test to confirm the presence of HIV-1 infection." So this is a HIV test that shouldn't be used as an HIV test. Confused?

Another one, Abbott Axsym HIV-1/HIV-2 test insert states: "At present there is no recognised standard for establishing the presence or absence of antibodies to HIV-1 and HIV-2 in human blood." So this test is for testing something, but actually the manufacturer doesn't know what it's testing for.

So how do HIV tests get you a certain result? There are two different types: the ELISA and the Western Blot. The first one is usually used first and the second one is only for verification in case the first one is positive. Both tests use HIV proteins, whatever they are. For as the manufacturers of the tests indicate, they don't know what they are testing for exactly. The ELISA is reasonably straightforward and inconclusive results can be turned positive or negative based on your answers on the questionnaire. The Western Blot is a bit more complicated, as it works with multiple proteins. But the basics are the same. And what exactly is positive or negative depends on a variety of factors. One is the brand of test. As the results need to be interpreted the manufacturer of the test gives instructions how to interpret and this can be different per brand. So the exactly same blood sample can be positive with one brand and negative with another. The second is the lab assistant who does the interpreting. They are humans and might interpret your questionnaire in a certain way and give you the benefit of the doubt, or not. The third one depends on the country that you live in. The Western Blot test uses multiple proteins, so you can be positive for one and negative for another. In some countries you are positive with just one or two markers. On the other hand, in other countries you need four or even five markers to be positive. So if you have a positive test in the USA all you need to do is move to Australia with the same test result and at once you are negative.

And of course you think that at least with a positive test you have a dangerous infection or your health is otherwise at risk. After all, you have a positive test result for something. Again, this is a no. It is known that a variety of situations can cause a positive HIV test. Long lists of conditions exist and it goes from pregnancy and flu to stress and nutrient deficiencies. Pretty much anything can cause a positive test. Two weeks later your test might be negative.

This should shock everyone. But what worries me the most is not the laughable test procedures, but the fact that these tests are generally used all over the world, with often far reaching consequences for those who get a positive result. How is it possible that neither doctors nor lab assistants blow the whistle? HIV testing is not science, it's not even quackery, it's a very dangerous hoax.

AIDS

As HIV testing is a useless activity, how is AIDS diagnosed? After all, even if you have a positive test result, this doesn't mean that you are sick. So what is AIDS? If asked many people will look puzzled, mention a few a symptoms and then admit that they don't know. Ask any doctor and they will give you the same reaction. The reason for this is that there is no definition of AIDS. AIDS is everything and anything, depending on the person, time and geographical location. AIDS in an American gay man is something totally different than AIDS in a German haemophiliac, which is something totally different than in an African woman, which is something totally different than in an Asian businessman. And the descriptions also change from time to time, whatever the political situation in any country requires. That's the reason why no doctor can tell you what AIDS looks like.

In certain regions in Africa it's recognised that the test is useless. These people carry a certain bacteria with them that gives an almost 100% positive test result. So they don't test. They use a list of symptoms (the Bangui clinical diagnosis of AIDS) to decide whether someone has AIDS. Different symptoms have different points and you need 12 points to have AIDS. Severe weight loss and weakness both score 4 points. Fevers and diarrhoea for more than a month give you both 3 points. Coughs and rashes also give points. These are symptoms of tuberculosis and malaria, diseases that happen to be very common in Africa. These diseases have been around for a very long time, but now at once these poor people are told that they have AIDS, with the horrible emotional, social and physical consequences. Being told that you have a fatal disease, then being kicked out of the community and not getting proper treatment for your real disease is enough to make people die within a year. The reason why this happens is mainly money. The WHO and rich countries won't give any money to get rid of poverty, malaria and tuberculosis. But an AIDS epidemic can get a country generous funding. When a country gets a new government that decides that they don't want that many people with AIDS they can simply abandon this way of diagnosing and at once there is no AIDS anymore. That's why the AIDS epidemic in Africa comes and goes.

Drugs
What about the anti-retroviral drugs? Don't they work? When the first AIDS patients were defined as such and HIV was appointed as the cause, drugs were of course demanded to treat the condition. The first one was Zidovudine, or azidothymidine, generally known as AZT. This drug had initially been developed as a chemotherapy drug, but it was too toxic and it ended up on the shelf. For reasons

that are hard to explain this same drug was at once decided to be effective against HIV and it became generally prescribed. Chemotherapy drugs are usually only given for short periods of time, for the stuff is so toxic that it would kill you if you take it for too long. Now a chemo drug that was classified as too dangerous for cancer got prescribed for daily use. And from that moment the AIDS patients started to drop dead everywhere. The official cause of death was AIDS, but it's not so hard to see that they died from the drug. Men who were perfectly healthy got a positive HIV test, started with AZT and were dead within a year. So drug poisoning can be put on the list of AIDS symptoms.

Quite a few other anti-retroviral drugs have since made it on the market. Some are less toxic than AZT, but most are about the same dangerous. The main problem is that they cause organ failure. Liver and heart diseases are very common among those taking anti-retrovirals. But also general wasting is a common one. Basically all the symptoms that are supposed to be caused by AIDS are also problems caused by the drugs. Many people are healthy when they get a HIV diagnosis and start taking these drugs. Soon they will start to get "AIDS" symptoms. But how can anyone know the difference between AIDS and drug poisoning when the problems are identical?

But it seems like some people who have been diagnosed with AIDS (not just HIV) do better after starting the drugs. The reason is that those people usually have bacterial infections as well. Anti-retrovirals prevent cells from multiplying. That works on the virus, on the body's own cells and also on bacteria. Without bacterial infection you will feel better, but the effect won't last long, as the drugs are too toxic.

And then there is the magic CD4 count. This is supposed to be above 200 and if it goes under that you are in trouble. When a person with a low CD4 count starts taking the drugs indeed usually the count goes up. The patient gets told that the virus responds well to the therapy. But the reality is that the CD4 count goes up in defence against the toxic drugs. After a while the immune system gets overwhelmed and the number goes down rapidly. "The virus has developed resistance against the drugs." In reality the body has been poisoned.

So let's have a look at the insert of these drugs, for there is something interesting to read. They all say something like "there is no proof that this drug will make you live longer". Huh? Isn't that the reason why people take them? Whoever take these highly toxic drugs do so because they think they will live longer than if they don't take it. How is it possible that these drugs are still on the market and that doctors still prescribe them? Well, that's the power of the pharmaceutical industry.

Summary

So here's a summary of the HIV/AIDS discussion. HIV has never been proven to cause disease. The test is not meant to be used to diagnose the infection. The disease symptoms are whatever is convenient. And the drugs that are given to treat the disease have no proof that they actually do that. Both HIV and AIDS are not just a hoax. They are a scam that has killed many.

13. Food

It's a big myth in itself that doctors know about food. They know close to nothing and what they know is usually wrong. Still they have no problem giving patients dietary advice. But sometimes they send the patient to the dietician. Dieticians of course know a lot more about food, as they have studied that for three years. But the problem is that after three years of study they still can't produce a lot of useful information. They have the habit of treating everyone as the standard. But have you ever met the standard person? And if you ask them questions beyond the standard things they have no idea what to say.

Fat is bad?
It is shocking how many doctors (and dieticians for that matter) still stick with the "fat is bad" and "fat makes you fat" myths. And the little bit of fat they do allow you to eat must be polyunsaturated, as that is so much healthier. None of this is remotely true. Let's first look at the idea that eating fat makes you fat. Both doctors and dieticians should know that fat gets digested and does not simply move to your hips or belly. The whole idea is too absurd. Slowly some of them start to realise that the idea is not correct, but it's still a common theory.
So is fat bad for you? Of course it's not! We need fat and a lot of it. Lots of nutrients can only be properly absorbed with fat. Eating a high fat diet is also good for diabetics, as fat doesn't influence blood sugar. It's actually good for everyone, as long as you eat good quality fats.

So there is the story about saturated fat being bad for your heart. When you look into that you quickly discover that this myth was based on fraudulent research. In the 1960's a guy named Ancel Keys had this idea that saturated fat causes high cholesterol and that this causes heart attacks. He collected all the information that was available, which included data from 22 countries. It appeared that the data were all over the place. People with high fat diets had high or low cholesterol and people with high cholesterol did or did not get heart attacks. A proper scientist at this moment comes to the conclusion that his theory was obviously wrong and throws the whole lot into the rubbish bin. But not so Ancel Keys. He simply threw out the data of 15 countries and published a "seven countries study". Those seven happened to show what he wanted, purely by chance. This is not science. This is fraud. Initially the guy had trouble to get this research published because it was so shoddy. But somehow at some point he managed to convince a group of important people that he didn't have time to do proper research, as in the meantime so many people would die from heart attacks. The logic was completely absent, but somehow this got accepted and from that moment we were stuck with the idea that we should eat a lot of vegetable oils. And from that moment the number of heart attacks started to increase rapidly. For heart attacks are not caused by cholesterol. The tissue that causes blocked arteries contains only a little bit of cholesterol. Its main cause is inflammation and most vegetable oils cause exactly that. Add a lack of vitamin C (which is remarkably common nowadays) and you have an explanation why heart attacks are one of the main causes of death in western countries.

If you want to know what e.g. canola oil is you can look that up on line. There are some interesting videos on YouTube, which first explain the stomach turning production process of these oils and then tell you how healthy this stuff is.

Carbohydrates

There are three types of nutritional and calorie sources: fat, protein and carbohydrates. It's funny how often you read that you shouldn't eat a lot of carbohydrates, but load up on fruit and vegetables. That's nonsense. Fruit and vegetables contain a lot of carbohydrates. The authors of such writings usually mean that you shouldn't eat a lot of grains and they have a point there. In contrast with mainstream nutritional advice grains are not an essential food group. You can be perfectly healthy without grains. The main reason why all over the world grains are a dietary staple is that it's easy. Fruit and vegetables go off easily, but when you properly store grains they can last a long time. Nevertheless you can very well do without them. Some people feel a lot better if they don't eat grains, but for most people they are not a problem.

Of course there are more and more people who have a gluten allergy. They can eat e.g. rice or corn, but must avoid many other grains. Doctors will tell you that the reason for the huge increase in gluten allergy is unknown. (They rarely know why there is such a huge increase in a variety of chronic and degenerative diseases.) There are a few things that stand out though. The wheat we eat nowadays is cultivated to contain a very high level of gluten, because this is so easy for the food industry. 200 years ago wheat was different. But still this doesn't quite explain the problem. Huge amounts of pesticides are used to grow wheat, which is necessary because soil depletion makes the crops sensitive to all kinds of pests. Doctors will tell you that the currently used pesticides are safe, as they are approved by the government. So were lead-arsenate, DDT and a variety of other highly toxic substances. You would expect doctors to understand that poison is unhealthy, but they usually don't. Then there is another cause, that is not very well known. Some vaccines are made with a gluten containing growth medium. Some of this growth medium likely will make it into the vaccine and injection of gluten will likely lead to a gluten allergy. It's probably just a little bit that ends up in a batch of vaccines, which could explain why not everyone gets a gluten allergy, just like not everyone gets a peanut allergy after being injected with a vaccine that is made with peanut oil. Likely not every vaccine contains a piece of the protein. Or maybe not everyone reacts to a tiny bit of protein with developing an allergy. It's hard to know, as nobody ever researches this.

Fruit and vegetables
Even doctors and dieticians know that fruit and vegetables are good for you. But the guidelines about how much you should eat of them are pretty absurd. For these guidelines assume that everyone is the same. No matter how old you are, what your exercise level is, what your body type is and whether you are sick or healthy, everyone should eat the same amounts of fruit and vegetables. In reality one serve of vegetables and a small piece of fruit might be enough for some (especially children), while others need ten times as much. So messages in the media about "only so few people eat the recommended amounts of fruit and vegetables" you better take with a grain of salt. If you stay away from junk food you will likely eat more fruit and vegetables anyway.

Another myth is that if you eat healthy your will get all the nutrients you need. But for a lot of foods this is not true. Grains, fruit and vegetables are generally grown as monoculture and this depletes the soil. Few farmers nowadays use manure to fertilise. They use artificial fertiliser, which has very limited nutrients. The problem is that even with depleted soil the crops usually grow quite well. They look good, but don't contain a lot of nutrients anymore. This can easily be proven. There are reliable tables of 80 years ago, which show how much of all kinds of minerals were in crops then. Most crops now contain 10-20% of those amounts. So without supplements you will likely be malnourished. Small, organic farmers often use crop rotation and that is much better for the soil. Those crops will likely be much healthier, but still won't be as good as they used to be.

Sugar
At least the medical establishment has realised that sugar is not a very healthy food, though in general they don't quite understand how bad the truckloads of sugar are. And they don't understand how addictive sugar is. And so another myth was born: you can eat sugar in moderation. That's a nice theory, but it doesn't work. We live in a world that is saturated with sugar. There is sugar in pretty much everything, even in meat products and snacks that traditionally used to be savoury. The food industry has made us addicted to sugar. And anyone who has been addicted to something knows that cutting down doesn't work. An alcoholic cannot drink socially and a smoker cannot just cut back on the number of cigarettes. Neither can you cut back on your sugar intake. You can do it for a while on pure will power, but you will constantly feel like you miss out and pretty soon you will find yourself in a café with a sugary drink and a large piece of cake. Just like with other addictions the only way to stop is to quit completely. You sometimes read that sugar addiction is worse than cocaine, but that's another myth. If you have prepared properly quitting sugar isn't too hard. In most cases within 2-3 weeks the sugar cravings are gone and you don't even want the cake anymore. And then it becomes easy. When the thought of sugar makes you feel "yuk", then you won't eat it, no matter how much is around. It's the only way to do it and it's highly recommended. For your body doesn't need sugar and doing without will make you feel a lot better. But if you tell your doctor that you have quit sugar you will likely get a comment that "it's not necessary to completely cut out sugar".

Ignore it. They don't know any better.

Protein

The ideas about protein are more consistent. Don't eat too much of it and animal protein is easier digested and of higher quality than most plant proteins. But that's a very general idea. Vegetarians have always existed and most can stay perfectly healthy without meat. So for many people meat is not an essential food. But there are also people who get sick if they don't get meat. The health care professionals don't know these things. If they are meat eaters they will likely tell you that meat is essential and if they are vegetarians they likely will tell you that you can do very well without meat. They just don't know that people have different nutritional needs. And if you want to try a vegan diet, don't even bother telling any of these people. They don't know anything about it and likely will just produce a lot of nonsense. If for whatever reason you want to eat only plant foods, then give it a try. Some people can stay healthy that way, but many get sick sooner or later. The best way is to just try and see if it works for you. But if you get sick and see a doctor, don't expect them to make the connection with your diet. You will have to do that yourself.

Information

So where should you get your nutritional information? Not from the health care professionals. Not from diet gurus either. And you better stay away from all kinds of food fads. There are truckloads of information on line, but it can be hard to distinguish the good from the bad. There are a few basic guidelines for this. First of all you should eat real food. If it comes in colourful boxes and has ingredients that you cannot even pronounce, then stay away from it. Eat organic if you can. But most of all: use your common sense. Think about how your great-grandparents ate. They had healthy diets. And try different approaches. Not every person stays healthy on the same diet.

And what about super foods? Some of them are indeed very nutritious, but they only work to supplement a healthy diet. For it's not just about eating healthy food, but just as much about staying away from junk food. If you give your body bad fuel, then adding good fuel is not going to give a great result.

14. Gynaecology and obstetrics

Because of pregnancy and childbirth the female reproductive organs are a lot more complicated than the male ones, so it's not so strange that doctors pay more attention to women than to men. But a lot of things go wrong in this area.
Obstetricians are doctors who specialise in pregnancy and childbirth. And here you have two things that should better not go together. Pregnancy is not a disease and doctors should not get involved unless there are real medical problems.

Women have given birth for as long as there have been humans. Pregnancy is a complicated process and loads of things can go wrong. As a result there have always been women who died as a result of giving birth. But that number is actually not remotely as high as modern doctors want women to believe. Midwives have always done a great job in delivering babies and in areas where there are no doctors available they still do this great job. When only midwives are involved complications happen and women die, but it's not that common. Things first go wrong when doctors get involved.

History
In the mid 1800's doctors decided that it was much better for women to give birth in hospitals, instead of at home with the assistance of only a midwife. This resulted in many thousands of women dying from childbed fever. Then dr. Ignaz Semmelweis found out that it was the doctors who spread the bacteria and if they would wash their hands the dreaded fever would disappear from the hospital. You would expect that the doctors would have been overjoyed with this finding, as now all these young mothers wouldn't need to die anymore. Nothing like that happened. The doctors couldn't stand the idea that they were responsible and dr. Semmelweis was ostracised. The doctors went on for more than 20 years causing childbed fever till hand washing finally became a standard practice.
You would think that this would have made clear that hospitals are not a good place to give birth and that doctors are not the ones you want to have around during that time. But somehow this message didn't get through and in many countries the hospital birth is the standard and home birthing is strongly discouraged, as it should be

too dangerous.

Interesting detail: in my home country, the Netherlands, for a very long time the home birth was the standard and insurance companies wouldn't even cover a hospital birth if there wasn't a medical reason for it. And till recently the obstetrician was an unknown profession. This didn't cause any problems whatsoever, but it did keep the percentage of interferences low. Unfortunately the medical system started to convince women that a hospital birth was safer and the percentage of home births has gone down to about 20%. And with that the percentage of c-sections and other birthing procedures has gone up.

Interference
So what do obstetricians do? From early in the pregnancy they do tests. Doctors love tests, no matter how useless they are. Pregnancy ultrasounds are standard in many countries and they are considered perfectly safe. This was also thought about pregnancy X-rays, till it appeared that these photos caused cancer in the children. It took doctors some 20 years before pregnancy X-rays were abandoned. A lot of evidence exists now that ultrasounds are not safe either, but it will likely take another 20 years before this practice will also be abandoned. Doctors are not eager to learn from their mistakes.

Depending on the country a lot of other tests are offered to women as soon as they are pregnant. As these tests are not very accurate many women are diagnosed with all kinds of problems that don't exist, or that solve themselves later during the pregnancy. But these problems result in more tests and more interference during the delivery. It's obvious that c-sections sometimes save lives. But the number is going extremely out of hand.
In Australia about 50% of the babies get born either by c-section or with other serious interference. 20% more in private than in public hospitals. The latter is a big red flag. Considering that risky pregnancies are a matter for public hospitals anyway you can only conclude that many c-sections are done for other than medical reasons.

The problem is that for the woman it's hard to know if she really needs an operation or other interference, or that the baby will come out on its own, without any problems. C-sections are pretty heavy operations, which can cause trauma and all kinds of physical problems. The idea that "it's just a c-section" is very far away from the truth. When women ask for a c-section for other than medical reasons doctors should strongly advise against it, or refuse to do it. That's the principle of "first do no harm", not even when the patient asks for it.

When the baby is born in hospital doctors and nurses are immediately around to interfere with everything. The cord gets clamped immediately (a dangerous procedure), the baby gets washed with toxic bathing products and sometimes it can take quite a while before mother and baby can start to get acquainted. I have no idea why anyone would think this is a good idea. In some countries the baby is left alone after that, but in other countries the needles come out immediately. The baby gets a shot with vitamin K and sometimes also a hepatitis B vaccine. It's a miracle that babies survive this.

Vitamin K
So what is it about the vitamin K? It sounds so innocent, but it's far from that. Besides it's completely unnecessary.

When a baby gets born this is a pretty violent process. Getting pushed through the birth canal is hard on the head and this causes loads of tiny bleeds in the baby's brain. That's perfectly normal and nothing to worry about. Nature has the perfect way to solve this problem. The cord blood is chockfull of stem cells and when these get into the baby they travel to the brain where they neatly repair any damage.

But what happened when doctors got involved in the birthing process? They decided that the cord had to be clamped immediately. As a result the stem cells don't get into the baby and can't do their important repair job. So babies started to get serious brain bleeds. Then doctors got the idea that vitamin K helps with blood clotting and they found out that babies have very low levels of vitamin K. And so they invented the vitamin K drops or injection for babies.

Why has a baby low vitamin K? Because if the blood would be too thick and clot too easily the stem cells couldn't travel to the brain. The blood must be this thin. So why do doctors get the idea that the low vitamin K is a flawed design? Eight days after birth the baby's blood clots well, which is the reason why Jews never circumcised before that day.

Babies are born with a perfect design and don't need any correction with pharmaceutical products.

Gynaecology

Also without a pregnancy doctors like to interfere with women's reproductive organs. The general rule "don't go to a doctor when you aren't sick" most definitely applies here. Many doctors love to find things that are wrong with women and start treating when there isn't a problem. Gynaecological exams are generally experienced by women as humiliating and they are rarely of any use.

Once menopause hits the doctors get really busy. Menopause is not a disease and shouldn't be treated as such. Most menopausal problems can actually be solved with a change in diet, but doctors don't know about diets and usually don't care. So they prescribe drugs. Hormone replacement therapy is a common one, like lack of oestrogen is a disease. It's known that this comes with all kinds of health risks, but that doesn't stop doctors from prescribing these synthetic hormones. And unfortunately many women also ask for the drugs, as they have been conditioned to think that a drug is better than changing your lifestyle.

Middle age comes with all kinds of issues and quite a few women end up in the office of a gynaecologist. And it's shocking how often it's quickly suggested that a hysterectomy would be the solution. This is major surgery, but doctors like to talk about it like it's no big deal. In the USA more than 30% of the women above 60 years old have got their uterus removed. In Australia it's even a bit higher. There is absolutely no justification for this. No doubt there are cases where a hysterectomy is the only way to solve problems, but it's shocking how easily doctors cut women open. And hysterectomy means removal of the uterus, but in many cases the ovaries are removed as well, often without the woman even knowing about this. The justification that is given is that removing the ovaries takes away the chance for ovarian cancer, which is considered difficult to treat. And it's not like a woman doesn't need her ovaries anymore after menopause. The ovaries keep producing hormones, so without them a woman can expect health problems. So the doctor prescribes synthetic hormones.

That still leaves out the issue that a woman without her reproductive organs might not feel like a woman anymore, even if she is past childbearing age. But the psychological component of medical treatments is generally ignored by doctors and it's not any different with this.

Removal of all the female reproductive organs is a castration. Many women would think twice about the surgery when they would know this. Men don't want to be castrated and neither do women.

The pill
That leaves the issue of the oral contraceptive pill. That's a difficult one. It's known that these pills are unhealthy and can cause all kinds of problems. The pill has been available now for more than 50 years and loads of new ones have been invented all the time. The newer ones cause even more issues than the older ones, but synthetic hormones are unhealthy. On the other hand it's obvious that the pill is very easy. So every woman needs to decide for herself whether it's a good idea to use it. But never rely on your doctor for proper information. Also with this doctors have no idea.

An extra warning is in place for teenage girls. Though many teenagers have sex and teenage pregnancy is not a desirable situation, it's a fact that these young girls have not fully developed yet. Also their hormones still need to mature and interfering with that process with synthetic hormones is a recipe for disaster. Doctors generally won't warn them for that. But they should, as teenagers cannot oversee the long-term health effects. And parents are not always involved in the decision. It's difficult to know how to solve this problem, when doctors don't do their job.

Conclusion

This book is not remotely complete. It's meant to make you think about the different topics and to encourage you to do more research. My goal was to make you realise that modern medicine is not "evidence based", but is largely based on assumptions and fantasies.

The best medical advice I can give is to never blindly trust a doctor. History and present have made clear that medical treatments do a lot more harm than good, so in general it's best to stay away from doctors. But if you choose to use the services of a medical practitioner for yourself or your loved ones, always keep a critical eye on what is done. If you can do some research before agreeing to a treatment. Doctors think that they know a lot about the human body, but in reality they have barely scratched the surface. And that shows in what they are doing.

Whatever you choose, keep in mind: "Don't trust me, I'm a doctor". It might save your life.